CANCER – NOT MY STORY

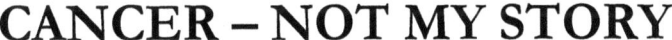

First Printing: August 2012
ISBN #: 978-1-105-74112-8

Table of Contents

Foreword

„If you don't look after yourself, life will be a song which you may never hear"
Unknown source

According to American Cancer Society 1.6 million people will be diagnosed with cancer in USA in 2012. That is 0,5% of total population. Multiply that with average 75 years lifespan and we come to breathtaking figure of 120 million people (40% of total population[1]) diagnosed with cancer in merely 75 years in USA alone! These are current trends and this is our reality. Some argue that this kind of wholesale cancer epidemic could not have happened by accident.

I dedicate this booklet to all in need of care, who wait for their magic „cure" which always seems around the corner… but never arrives on time. Or it may exist but patient is not aware of it. Because cancer really is an adverse opponent, one that lurks in the shadows, waiting patiently for you to let your guard down and striking while you sleep. Many have lost this battle, not because they didn't fought bravely and valiantly once the menace struck but because they even didn't see it coming. Fortunately though, there are remedies even for those who took their time with cancer diagnosis.

---

[1] not accounting for population growth

Introduction

This book has three main objectives. One is to portray a broader picture of causes that can ultimately lead to cancer development. And there are two schools of thought. One if official and regards cancer as "uncontrollable tissue growth". Other is unofficial where most proponents of alternative medicine view cancer or "uncontrollable tissue growth" not as start of something but rather as a result of parasite infection.

Second objective is to describe some natural and cheap ways to prevent and treat cancer. There are again two schools of thought. "Official" sticks strictly to standard practices of surgery, radiation and chemotherapy. "Unofficial" one is looking at root and cause of the problem, mostly wrong diet, lack of enzymes, insufficient oxygenation, acidic body etc.

Third objective is overall awareness raising of what people should be conscious of in their daily lives not to be surprised by possible "blitzkrieg" which may come. For beginning it is important to understand that cancer prevention is not a guarantee for bullet proof health but rather a question of risk management. Fortunately, you can manage this risk somewhat easily and cheaply - and sooner you start the better.

According to GLOBOCAN[2] 7.6 million cancer deaths and 12.7 million cancer cases are estimated to have occurred in 2008. 56% of the cases and 64% of the deaths occurred in the economically developing world. Breast cancer is the most frequently diagnosed cancer and the leading cause of cancer death among females, accounting 14% of the cancer deaths and lung cancer is the leading cancer site in males, totaling 23% of the total cancer deaths in 2008 estimate[3] . This makes invasive cancer the leading cause of death in the developed world and the second leading cause of death in the developing world. Over half of cases occur in the developing world. According to World Health Organization, however, it causes about 12.5% of all deaths worldwide[4] .

---

[2] Cancer Incidence, Mortality and Prevalence Worldwide in 2008; http://globocan.iarc.fr/

[3] CA: A Cancer Journal for Clinicians, volume 61, Issue 2 (April 2011)

[4] WHO report on cancer, 2007

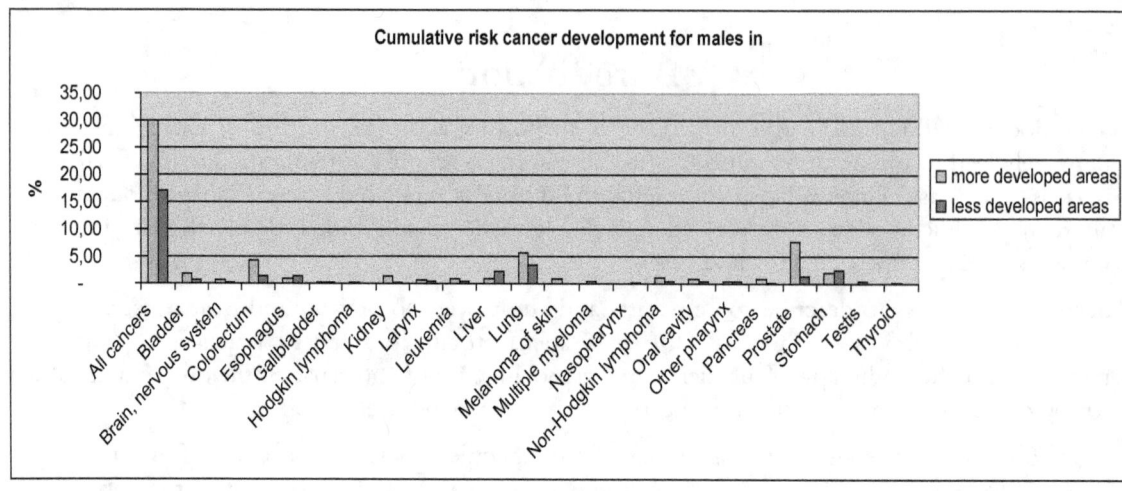

Source: A Cancer Journal for Clinicians, volume 61, Issue 2 (April 2011)

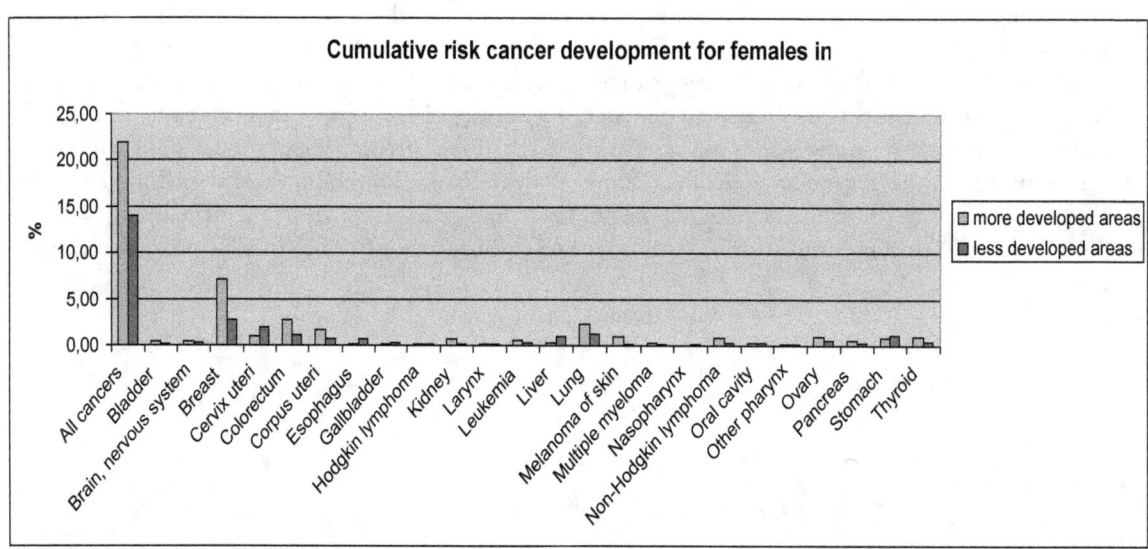

Source: A Cancer Journal for Clinicians, volume 61, Issue 2 (April 2011)

Faced with this onslaught doctors and pharmaceuticals seemed helpless for years. Not least because it's a simple thing to unravel but because it is polymorph with many faces and values, constantly changing and dependant of many variables, seemingly striking it's victims on sample basis. There are no certain rules pointing when disease will develop in human beings[5] or, more importantly when not! So it is important to watch out as 1$ worth of prevention brings more value than 100$ worth of treatment ! For example several studies have connected chlorinated

---

[5] as opposite to laboratory induced cancer on test animals

water to breast and colon cancer. Installing a simple graphite water filter worth 10$ is will certainly relieve you of that worry. Or exposure to harmful UV rays causes melanoma all over the world. Simply avoiding exposure to sun at critical hours doesn't cost anything !

Mortality from All cancers
Age-standardised rate (World), Male all ages

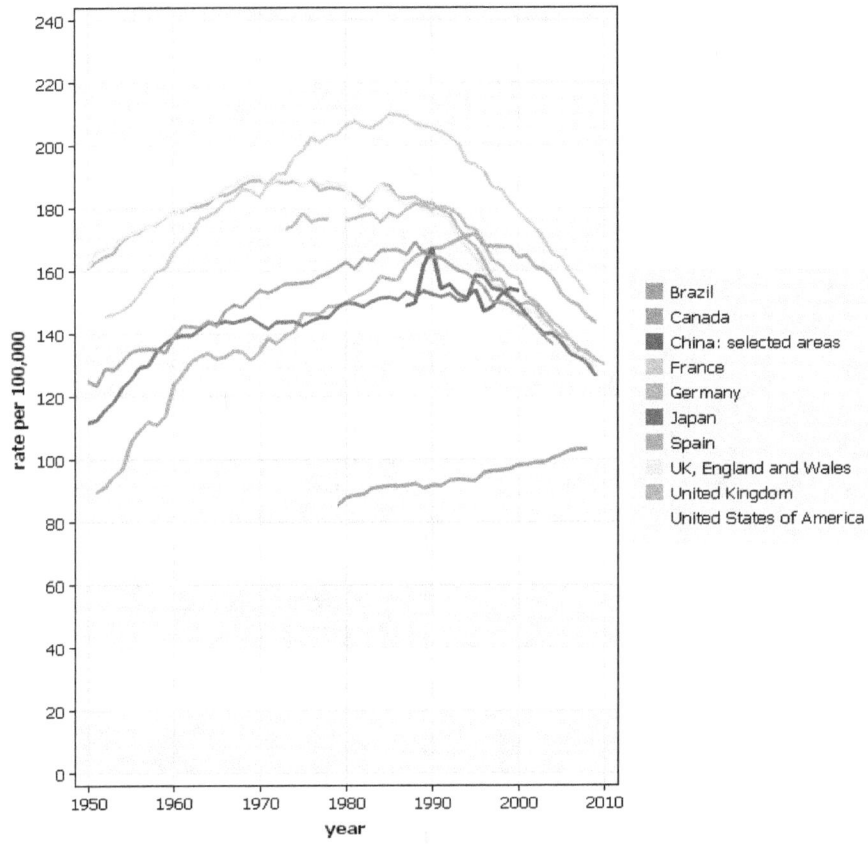

International Agency for Research on Cancer (IARC) - 1.3.2012

Source: WHO; http://www-dep.iarc.fr/

Trend in last 30 years gives rise to some optimism as "Age standardized rate" of cancer death seems to be slightly falling which means we already reached peak of these "plague" and situation overall is slightly improving, at least as surviving rates are concerned. Fortunately many cancer cases can be successfully treated if detected on time and prevention is something that helps this statistics.

So, number of people cured from particular type of cancer is rising, or to say it otherwise average number of deaths per 100.000 citizens is falling - meaning that all those billions pored in research&development of new drugs and treatments might give some results. Although alternative practitioners would have something to say about this.

Unfortunately, this is in contradiction to fact that number of people developing cancer is also rising. So more people are developing cancer but there are fewer deaths from it.

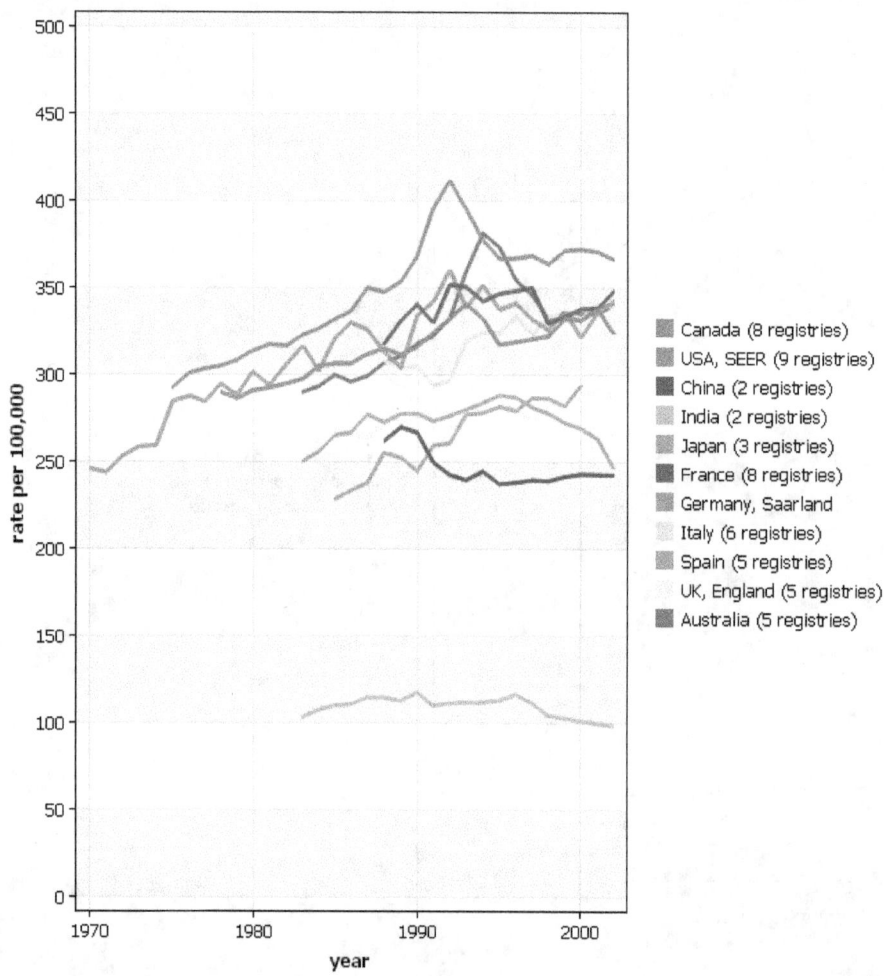

All sites but non-melanoma skin
Age Standardised Incidence Rate (World), Male age [0-85+]

International Agency for Research on Cancer (IARC) - 1.3.2012

Source: International Agency for Cancer Research; http://ci5.iarc.fr/CI5plus/ci5plus.htm

But this however should not give rise to extreme optimism. Down side is that cancer treatments may be unavailable to average human being for at least 2 reasons. One is that if someone lives in 3rd world country where technology itself is not available and other is of course, money ie.

treatments and drugs cost money even if they are available. Without 1st rate insurance policy chance is rather slim everyone will be able to obtain purposeful medical help. But bare in mind 1$ today is worth 10$ in six months so if there are any chances of somebody paying for expansive treatments its better to try to obtain funds as soon as disease was detected. Because, later it will be several times more expansive if cancer indeed develops and metastases occur.

This terrible and selfish flashback to materiality of our world all the more shows the importance of manning the defenses yourself before it's too late as not become impoverished afterwards.

Not to underestimate the size of our menace or its treacherous nature, unfortunately there are already signs that cancer related adverts for food stuffs or supplements are appearing on TV (like ORAC[6] scale, antioxidants, free radicals) to make money for it's producers. So we as society decided to make profit on cancer cases. These can be disorienting and confusing drawing away patient's attention from more powerful methods of cure. We must bear in mind that no marketing tricks should undermine our desire and instinct to take personal and decisive steps in order to help ourselves.

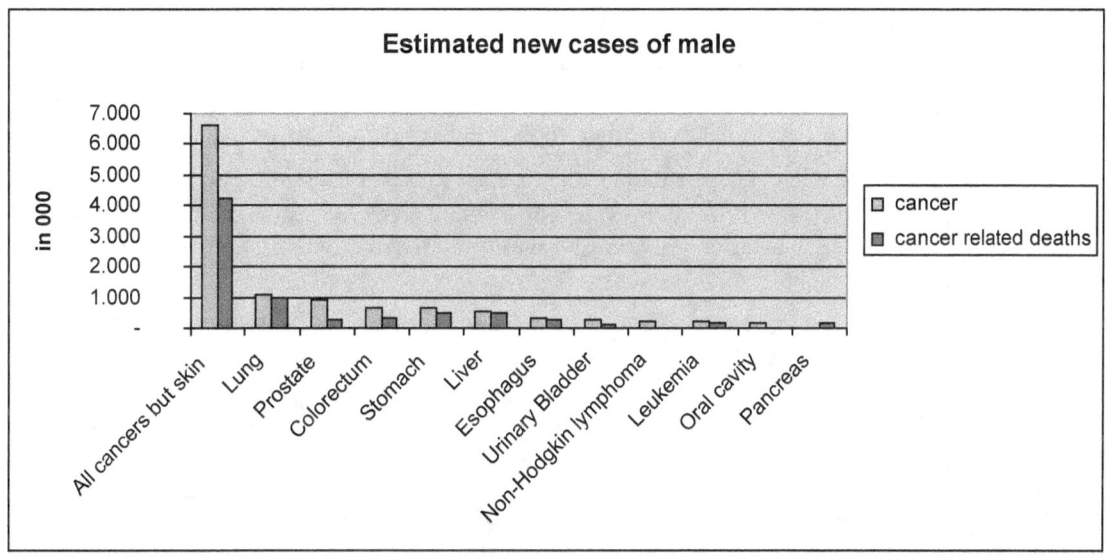

Source: CA: A Cancer Journal for Clinicians, volume 61, Issue 2 (April 2011)

---

[6] Oxygen Radical Absorbance Capacity - one of the most sensitive and reliable methods for measuring antioxidant capacity

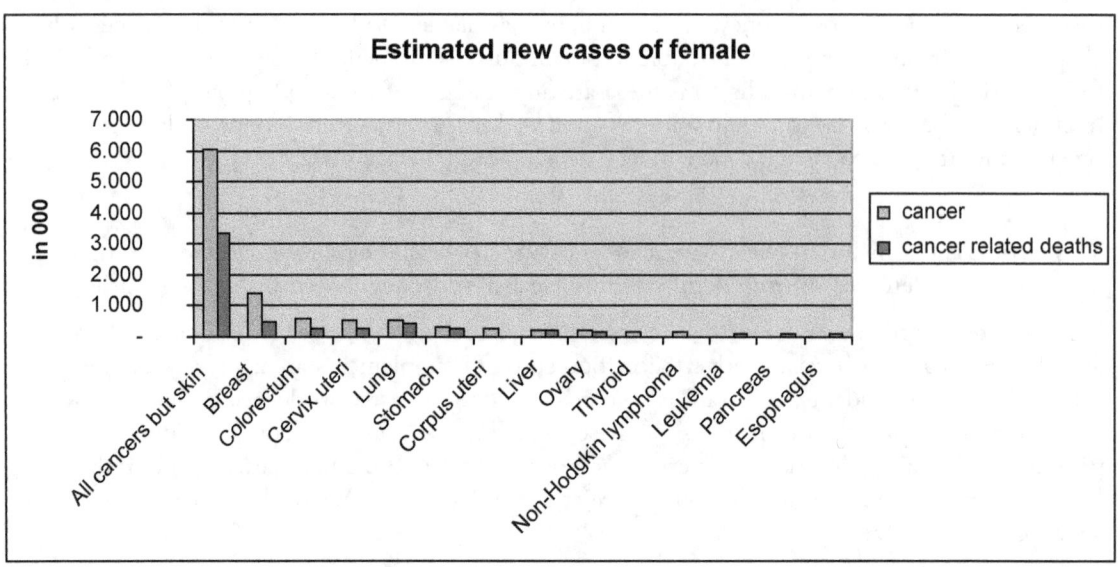

Source: CA: A Cancer Journal for Clinicians, volume 61, Issue 2 (April 2011)

No all cancers should be made in same breath. Some are more lethal than others. Melanoma, for example, is lethal in more than 90% of time if it reaches IV stage of development. We can say that cancers that have bigger propensity for metastasis are more dangerous than others.

In a effort to understand what is happening we might need to travel back in time a bit. Obviously, not so long ago, let's say 1800 -1900 there were not so many cases of registered cancer patients. Something has obviously changed in meantime. If we shortly analyze what has changed we come to following things:

a) nature of work has changed, meaning less physical work which is generally good and more

   brain work (which often includes bad stress)

b) living environment has changed where more and more people are clogged in relative small

   space in cities

c) exposure to sun influence has decreased as we work more in offices and harmful UV rays are more potent than before due to destruction of ozone layer

d) air pollution has risen significantly, especially in cities

e) electrical&magnetic pollution has introduced significantly, especially in cities

f) food stuffs has moved from domestic to highly processed with lots of pesticides, antibiotics and preservatives of all kinds

g) vaccination and medicaments has been introduced widely, often consumed without prescription and supervision

h) drinking water got saturated with chemicals, namely harmful chlorine and fluoride

i) lifestyle changed as job security has decreased, workload increased alongside associated stress

Roughly we can summarize all of these into 3 categories:

a) things which we digest have changed

b) we became relieved of physical exercise and sunlight which degenerates our immune system (especially lymph which requires physical exertion in order to function properly)

c) we became exposed to all sorts of various hazardous external influence like radiation and virus infections that did not exist before

One proof that these changes are very relevant to cancer is that Asians have been shown to have a 25 times lower incidence of prostate cancer and a ten times lower incidence of breast cancer than do residents of Western countries. However, rates for these cancer casses increased substantially after Asians migrated to the West (presumably because they encountered different living conditions[7]).

We need no brainstorming to instinctively know that aforementioned things are bad for us.

Million dollar question is just **how bad** ?

And **why** do they obviously induce all sorts of malignant diseases ?

And **what** to do to protect ourselves?

---

[7] Anand, Preetha, Kunnumakara, Ajaikumar, et al. (2008). Cancer is a preventable Disease that Requires Major Lifestyle Changes

I. Possible causes of cancer

The important thing here is to understand at least roughly what is happening, how aforementioned categories influence our organism and why we can succumb to disease. "Offical" medicine says that cancer pathogenesis is traceable back to DNA mutations that impact cell growth and metastasis. Substances that cause DNA mutations are known as mutagens, and mutagens that cause cancers are known as carcinogens.

Cancers are primarily an environmental disease with 90-95% of cases attributed to environmental factors (radiation, food, stress) and 5-10% due to genetics. Environmental, as used by cancer researchers, means any cause that is not genetic. Common environmental factors that contribute to cancer death include tobacco (25-30%), diet and obesity (30-35%), infections of all kinds (15-20%), radiation (both ionizing and non-ionizing, up to 10%), stress, lack of physical activity, and environmental pollutants etc.[8].

It must be said here that these factors are usually self-amplifying meaning for example that stress decreasses our immune system and we are more prone to cancer development induced by radiation, viruses etc. So, although one factor is prevailing it usually takes more to do us in.

Cell duplication and fuel

Let's say our body consists of billions of little cells usually several microns in diameter. These little cells form tissues and tissues form organs. In 1 cubic millimeter there can be a million cells. Cells came to life with cell duplication meaning existing cells divide and then new cells also divide and that is how we grow. Particular type of cells grow at different rate, so for example hair, skin, fingernails, taste buds, and the stomach's protective lining are replaced constantly and at a rapid rate throughout our lives. This is in contrast to nerve cells in the central nervous system are rarely produced after we are a few months old.

This process of cell duplication is no "perpetum mobile" by any stretch of imagination, meaning cells require, among other things, "fuel" of sufficient quality to grow, work and divide. Without "fuel" of particular quality this process will not be normal and ill may we become. Our body is not what it thinks of itself but what it consumes. If junk is what you eat, junk is what will grow eventually. Simple as that.

Another example of what can go wrong could be that aforementioned hazardous external influence that can damage existing cells DNA which in turn losses ability to replicate correctly, meaning new cells are no replicas of old cells so instead of having one "damaged" cell to start with we have two after division etc.

---

[8] "Cancer is a Preventable Disease that Requires Major Lifestyle Changes";Preetha Anand, Ajaikumar B. Kunnumakara, Chitra Sundaram, Kuzhuvelil B. Harikumar, Sheeja T. Tharakan, Oiki S. Lai, Bokyung Sung, and Bharat B. Aggarwal

Oxygen&ph&sugar

There are also studies suggesting that lower pH values (below 7) severely affect carcinogen processes. Central point of this theory is a fact that only incremental movements on pH scale affect ability of blood to carry oxygen which is also know as Bohr effect[9].

A 0.1 difference in pH gives 10 times more or less negative hydrogen ions in blood, and .2 increments means 100 more or less hydrogen ions as well as reduced capability to transfer oxygen. Some researchers suggest that at pH of 7.4 cancer cells become dormant.

When starved of oxygen, cell mitochondria designated to produce energy by combining glucose and oxygen becomes irretrievably damaged. These cells loose their ability to produce energy correctly (naturally) and instead start to produce energy by fermenting sugar without much oxygen. This in turn produces lots of lactic acid in cancer cells.

Dr. Warburg and other scientists found was that respiratory enzymes in cells, which make energy aerobically using oxygen, die when cellular oxygen levels drop. For this he was awarded in 1931 Nobel Prize.

Poor oxygenation can come from several sources like from toxins which we eat, inhale or which occur in badly functioning colon. Toxins can damage cellular oxygen respiration mechanism. When this happens, the cell can no longer produce energy aerobically. So, if the cell is to live, it must, at least partially, ferment sugars, producing energy without oxygen. Fermentation allows these cells to survive, but they can no longer perform any functions in the body or communicate effectively with the body. Consequently, these cells can only multiply and grow.

What is striking is that cancer cells have 10-15 times more insulin receptors than normal cells. Having so much more insulin receptors than normal cells means that the effect of administered insulin will be ten times greater on cancer cells than on normal cells ie. they will also absorb far more glucose from blood.

It is a well-known scientific fact that cancer cells have a voracious appetite for glucose. Glucose is their unique source of energy, and because of the relatively inefficient way cancer cells burn this fuel, they use up a great deal of it. This is one reason why cancer patients lose so much weight. Because cancer cells require so much glucose, they virtually steal it away from the body's normal cells, thus starving them. The interesting connection between cancer cells and insulin is that recent findings published in the scientific medical literature report that cancer cells actually manufacture and secrete their own insulin[10].

---

[9] http://en.wikipedia.org/wiki/Bohr_effect

[10] http://www.contemporarymedicine.net/ipt_chemo.htm

Radiation

You also need to be aware of are hazardous external sources which include but are not limited to all kind of radiation (electric, magnetic, ionizing, non-ionizing), virus infections which -ultimately- result in irreparable DNA damage which can cause cancerous mutations further down the line. Radiation will be elaborated in more detail afterwards but for now it's enough to say is that it is all around us and has increased since humans discovered electricity and nuclear energy and generally speaking it can't be avoided entirely.

Even if you would to crawl in most distinct cave you can not escape nuclear fallout from detonated bombs and blown up reactors. Suffice to say is that this kind of radiation is called ionizing radiation and it works by damaging DNA through highly charged particles like alpha, betta, gamma particles etc.

Other kind of radiation is called non-ionizing and is thought to merely transit energy via it's long wavelengths but that is still open to discussion as for example high voltage electric current, although in low frequency field, can still be present as mutagen.

And yet another kind of radiation is present eternally and by those I mean geopathogen points, Hartman and Curry lines and such alike which are induced by planet Earth and universe itself. This kind of radiation is known to exist for long time and to be quite harmful but it is not nearly researched enough so it is somewhat covered by a veil of mist. Dr. Hartman however made a very firm connection between so called Hartman crosses and cancer patients.

There is also third "player" in this game of life and death and that is our immune-system.

Immune system

The idea behind immune system is that it targets foreign "intruders" that trigger response from immune system or recycles used up cells and debris in body. This "intruders" are also known as antigens. They can be a foreign cell, a bacterium, a virus, an MHC marker protein or even a portion of a protein from a foreign organism[11].

And this is where our immune system kicks in. Human immune system actually consists of:

- **Lymphocytes** are a type of white blood cell found in the blood and many other parts of the body. Types of lymphocytes include B cells, T cells, and Natural Killer cells.

  B cells (B lymphocytes) mature into plasma cells that secrete proteins called antibodies (immunoglobulins). Antibodies recognize and attach to foreign substances known as antigens, fitting together much the way a key fits a lock.

---

[11] National Cancer Institute; http://www.cancer.gov/cancertopics/understandingcancer/immunesystem/page1

Each type of B cell makes one specific antibody, which recognizes one specific antigen.

T cells (T lymphocytes) work primarily by producing proteins called cytokines. Cytokines allow immune system cells to communicate with each other and include lymphokines, interferons, interleukins, and colony-stimulating factors. Some T cells, called cytotoxic T cells, release pore-forming proteins that directly attack infected, foreign, or cancerous cells. Other T cells, called helper T cells, regulate the immune response by releasing cytokines to signal other immune system defenders.

Natural Killer cells (NK cells) produce powerful cytokines and pore-forming proteins that bind to and kill many foreign invaders, infected cells, and tumor cells. Unlike cytotoxic T cells, they are poised to attack quickly, upon their first encounter with their targets.

- **Phagocytes** are white blood cells that can swallow and digest microscopic organisms and particles in a process known as phagocytosis. There are several types of phagocytes, including **monocytes**, which circulate in the blood, and **macrophages**, which are located in tissues throughout the body.

The organs of immune system are positioned throughout human body. They are called lymphoid organs because they are home to lymphocytes--the white blood cells that are key operatives of the immune system. Within these organs, the lymphocytes grow, develop, and are deployed.

- *Bone marrow*, the soft tissue in the hollow center of bones, is the ultimate source of all blood cells, including the immune cells.

- The *thymus* is an organ that lies behind the breastbone; lymphocytes known as T lymphocytes, or just T cells, mature there.

- The *spleen* is a flattened organ at the upper left of the abdomen. Like the lymph nodes, the spleen contains specialized compartments where immune cells gather and confront antigens.

In addition to these organs, clumps of lymphoid tissue are found in many parts of the body, especially in the linings of the digestive tract and the airways and lungs--gateways to the body.

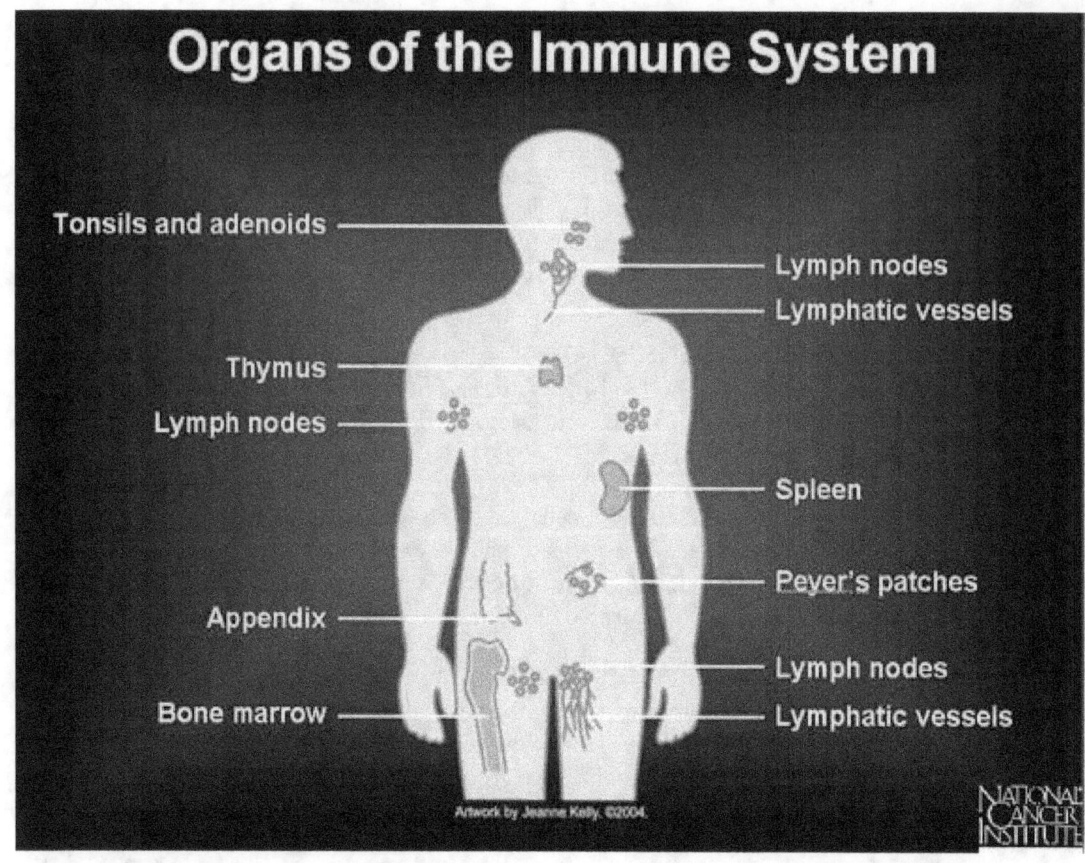

Source: The website of the National Cancer Institute (http://www.cancer.gov)

The organs of your immune system are connected with one another and with other organs of the body by a network of lymphatic vessels.

Lymphocytes can travel throughout the body using the *blood vessels*. The cells can also travel through a system of *lymphatic vessels* that closely parallels the body's veins and arteries. Cells and fluids are exchanged between blood and lymphatic vessels, enabling the lymphatic system to monitor the body for invading microbes. The lymphatic vessels carry *lymph*, a clear fluid that bathes the body's tissues[12]. Lymph requires exercise to work properly as it does not have central pump like heart in case of vascular system.

Benefits of exercise

Unfortunately evolution and genetics did not intend all to have excellent immune systems. Some people have weak immune system that is not so quite able to combat infections for example and to ultimately help repair the damage. But fortunately there are techniques that stimulate immune systems for better performance. For example regular exercises which increase heart beat rate help your body to better vent itself up of accumulated bad toxins and beef up immune systems.

---

[12] National Cancer Institute; http://www.cancer.gov/cancertopics/understandingcancer/immunesystem/page1

Current research seems to back this story up. Dr. Beth Levine and colleagues from University of Texas proved that exercise stimulate a process called "autophagy" which roughly means recycling used up and damaged parts of cells[13]. Via this process in human body, surplus, worn and malformed proteins are broken up and recycled. Autophagy also gains momentum when organism begins to starve and is relinquished of protein intake. Autphagy synthesizes amino-acid for cellular growth but these amino-acids can be also used for energy. Physical inactivity is believed to contribute to cancer risk not only through its effect on body weight but also through negative effects on immune system and endocrine system. Normal exercise (running) of 30 min. every couple of days should suffice and increase level of your immune system. Fitting is the quote from Frederick the Great, King of Prussia, claiming the "physical labor cures all ills".

It is also interesting to analyze "autophagy" process and rapid cancer growth as similar forces that deplete body weight. Whereas autophagy works by dissolving needless organelles in body when starving in order to survive, cancer in most cases devours protein mass to fuel it's rapid growth. Therefore autophagy logic probably does not work anymore when cancer starts growing rapidly as it is unlikely to stop it at this point. So extreme starvation is probably not likely to help with advanced cancer cases, it may work best in prevention.

These seem to support common stories in Europe of alive ww2 veterans who were serving on Russian front several years and lived to old age regardless of being Wehrmacht soldiers or partisans. They were obviously exposed to severe cold for quite and learned to survive on small rations [14]. This is in line with old but tried Victorian trick of boosting immune system is from being exposed to coldness for short periods of time. It is beneficial to go to cold places from time to time. You may get flue but your immune system will appreciate it. It is natural thing.

Pillars of health

Having in mind what was said about cell growth and duplication, hazardous damage to cells from foreign sources (viruses, radiation) and role play of our immune system we come to concept of Three Pillars of Health. These are so important they are written with capital letters and shown on following graph.

---

[13] Autophagy in Infection and Immunity; Beth Levine, Tamotsu Yoshimori, Vojo Deretic

[14] Of course only the toughest survived the harsh conditions to tell the tale

THREE PILLARS OF HEALTH

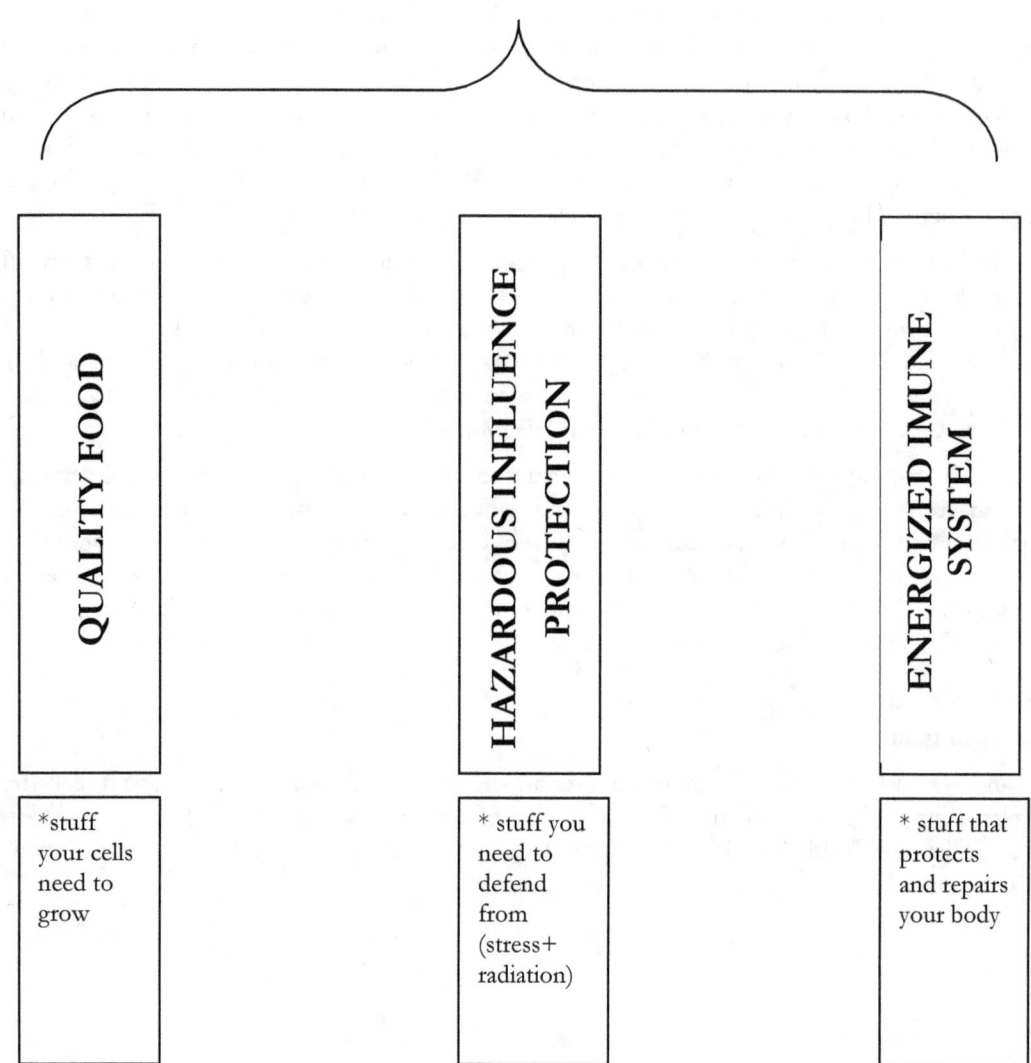

QUALITY FOOD

*stuff
your cells
need to
grow

**HAZARDOUS INFLUENCE
PROTECTION**

* stuff you
need to
defend
from
(stress+
radiation)

**ENERGIZED IMUNE
SYSTEM**

* stuff that
protects
and repairs
your body

End of the beginning

That brings us to conclusion that our cells can become malignant in three ways. First is our food consumption is so bad that cells don't receive anywhere near enough quality "fuel" they require (for example omega 3 fatty acids, alongside many other nutrients, are hugely important for healthy cell membranes) and malignant processes are therefore only question of time. Moreover, wrong kind of "fuel" can have disastrous consequences which will be further elaborated in next chapter. By fuel I mean also oxygen supply which partly depends on pH level of our body.

Second is that healthy cells can be rendered not only impotent but also malignant by process of outside influence usually electric/magnetic/nuclear radiation, chronic inflammation, particular virus infections, stress induced body reactions, genetic pre-determination etc.

And third is that cancer development depends on our immune system as well. There are things that boost the immune system like feasting and exercise and there are things which inhibit it like excess sugar consumption (which reduces vitamin C absorption by cells), physical inactivity etc.

1. Hazardous influence
-radiation&infections-

As previously mentioned one of the reasons why malignant cells occur is damage caused from external sources. Every material when put under sufficient stress - breaks. The question is just how much stress. Even iron and steel products break because of "material wear" meaning they will not last forever just because something is made of steel. And iron atoms don't replicate and regenerate themselves. Human cells do that, meaning human body is in somewhat better position to repair itself - to an extent. There is a measure for everything.

Statistics show that up to 10% of total cancer cases may be induced by radiation[15], both ionizing and nonionizing, like ultraviolet light (UV). Cancers induced by radiation include some types of leukemia, lymphoma, thyroid cancers, skin cancers, sarcomas, lung and breast carcinomas. Sweden experienced increased incidences of cancer cases after Chernobyl explosion. There are other sources of ionizing radiation like appliance of x-rays in medicine. *In fact, the risk of breast cancer from x-rays is highest among girls exposed to chest irradiation at puberty, a time of intense breast development*[16].

Ionizing radiation hits cells randomly. If it hits a chromosome or particular molecules in gene it can break the chromosome or inactivate one or more genes in the part of the chromosome that it hit. When major damage occurs the cell usually dies as part of programmed preventive measure. Smaller damage however may leave a cell open to further proliferating and ultimately cancer development, especially if tumor suppressor genes were damaged by the radiation.

As said earlier radiation from various sources covers entire spectrum and is divided in two major areas: ionizing and non-ionizing.

---

[15] D. Belpomme, P. Irigaray, L. Hardell, R. Clapp, L. Montagnier, S. Epstein, and A. J. Sasco. The multitude and diversity of environmental carcinogens. Environ. Res.105:414–429 (2007)

[16] Cancer is a Preventable Disease that Requires Major Lifestyle Changes; Preetha Anand, Ajaikumar B. Kunnumakara, Chitra Sundaram, Kuzhuvelil B. Harikumar, Sheeja T. Tharakan, Oiki S. Lai, Bokyung Sung, and Bharat B. Aggarwal; http://www.ncbi.nlm.nih.gov/pmc/articles/PMC2515569/

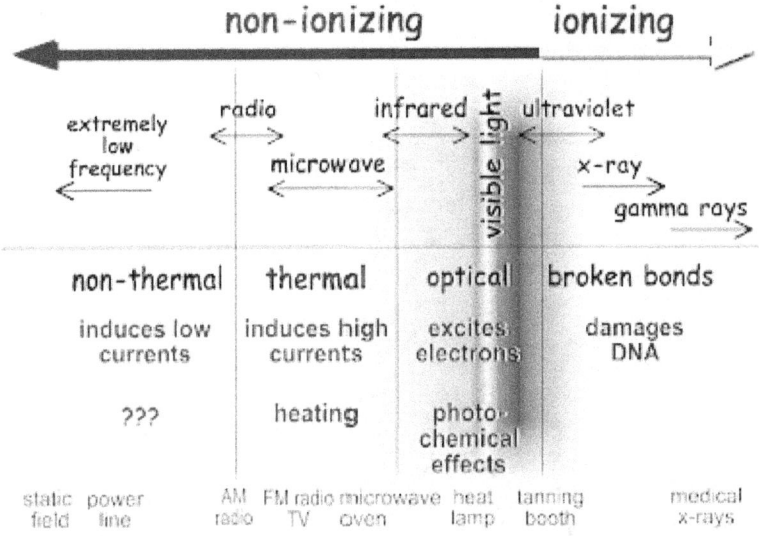

Source: http://en.wikipedia.org/wiki/Non-ionizing_radiation

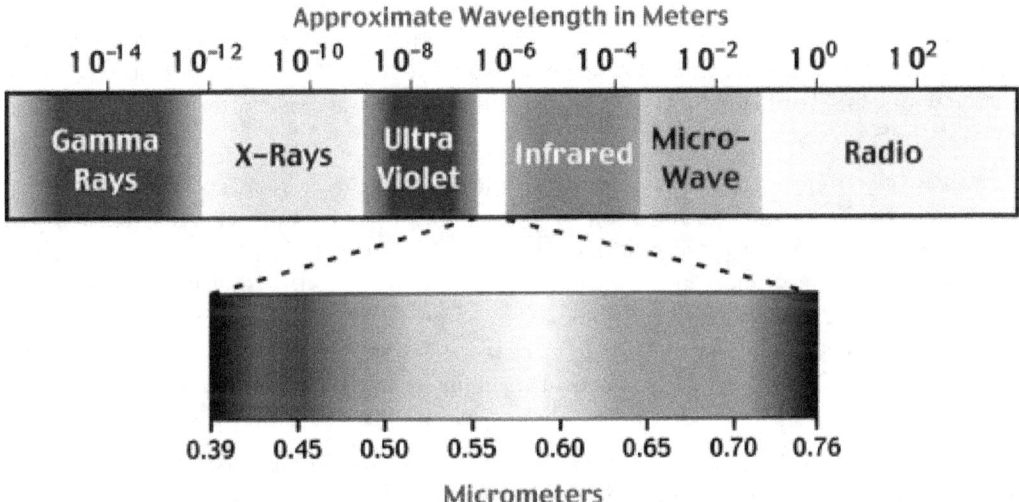

Radiation above is depicted via lengths of waves they emit. So gamma rays are extremely small in diameter ie. 100.000.000.000.000th part of 1 meter. And radio waves are more lengthy up to 100 meters in diameter.

First of all ions are just atoms that lost some electrons but to paint it simple ionizing radiation has enough energy to alter structures on molecular and atomic level meaning mutating your cells and if sufficient - causing cancer. X-rays and gamma-rays are considered ionizing radiation and quantity of allowed radiation is measured in miliSieverts[17]. We shall be more concerned here with electo&magnetic radiation and its measurements because it is far more common than ionizing radiation.

Nonionizing radiation derived primarily from sunlight includes UV rays, which in high quantity are carcinogenic to humans. Exposure to UV radiation is a major risk for various types of skin cancers including basal cell carcinoma, squamous cell carcinoma, and melanoma. Along with UV exposure from sunlight, UV exposure from sunbeds for cosmetic tanning may account for the growing incidence of melanoma.

Electrical and magnetic radiation are considered non-ionizing and in recent study International Agency for Research on Cancer[18] magnetic radiation from mobile phones classified as "possible carcinogenic". Electrical radiation occurs when current flows through conductor, like electrical wire. Usual measurement of electrical radiation is V/m or Volts per meter. According to American Council for Radiation Protection[19] threshold value for public is 10V/m at 50/60Hz. On top of above data showing length of waves there is also question of frequency of generating waves of particular length. And depending on frequency, threshold values for electric and magnetic radiation change as well. Therefore here are specified value for most common electricity running at 50/60 Hz.

Magnetic radiation occurs when current is being used or transformed in appliance like transformation, old TV sets, hairdryer, heaters etc…Measurement of magnetic radiation is mT or miliTesla and threshold value set by American Council for Radiation Protection for public is 0.04mT at 50/60Hz.

Low-frequency electromagnetic fields can cause clastogenic DNA damage. The sources of electromagnetic field exposure are high-voltage power lines, transformers, electric train engines, and more generally, all types of electrical equipments. An increased risk of cancers such as childhood leukemia, brain tumors and breast cancer has been attributed to electromagnetic field exposure. For instance, children living within 200 m of high-voltage power lines have a relative risk of leukemia of 69%, whereas those living between 200 and 600 m from these power lines have a relative risk of 23%. In addition, a recent meta-analysis of all available epidemiologic data showed that daily prolonged use of mobile phones for 10 years or more showed a consistent pattern of an increased risk of brain tumors[20].

The reason I put all those measurements is not because I expect all readers to understand them right away but to be aware that threshold values of electromagnetic radiation are set (but vary in each country quite widely) and you may have some sort of legal protection if those values in your home are exceeded.

---

[17] EPA annual limit of exposure to radiation for public

[18] http://www.iarc.fr/en/

[19] http://www.ncrppublications.org/index.cfm

[20] Cancer is a Preventable Disease that Requires Major Lifestyle Changes; Preetha Anand, Ajaikumar B. Kunnumakara, Chitra Sundaram, Kuzhuvelil B. Harikumar, Sheeja T. Tharakan, Oiki S. Lai, Bokyung Sung, and Bharat B. Aggarwal; http://www.ncbi.nlm.nih.gov/pmc/articles/PMC2515569/

Also good thing is that you can actually buy instruments that can measure electro&magnetic radiation in particular frequency range quite easily like the ones from Aaronia[21] for few hundred dollars, which if you think about it is not a bad investment. Especially if you are near high voltage power cable, underground trains etc. Or, alternatively, you can call in expert to do measurements for you.

With such instrument you can measure whether particular places in your apartment or house exceed threshold values, especially places you or your children spent lots of time in like bed, or learning table etc… If you happen to live in a city flat it is far more likely to be exposed to higher electromagnetic radiation than living in countryside house for example. Pay attention to electric sockets and power cables in walls, old TV, battery chargers etc. when looking for elevated radiation levels. After taking measurement I definitely decided to move my bad to better place as magnetic radiation was near threshold value.

Now when we talk about radiation we certainly must mention radiation coming from Earth by which I mean Hartmann and Curry lines. Earth radiates sort of magnetic radiation in several forms reason for which is still unknown. Most famous are Hartmann and Currry lines. German Doctor Hartmann discovered in 1951 that Earth surface is divided in sort of grid with longitude lines 2 meters apart and parallel lines 2.5 meters apart, but subject to change whether you are closer to poles or equator. Hartmann lines themselves are 21cm wide. They are everywhere even in each bedroom and in each bathroom. There is no effective way of stopping them. Needles to say spending huge amount of time on these lines is not good. Hartmann lines are almost lined up to Earths longitudes and latitudes meaning lines go north-south and east west deviating by 10 degrees. Especially bad are the crossings between these two directions of lines (N-S and E-W).

---

[21] http://www.spectran.com

This N-S and E-W grid an be visualized as follows:

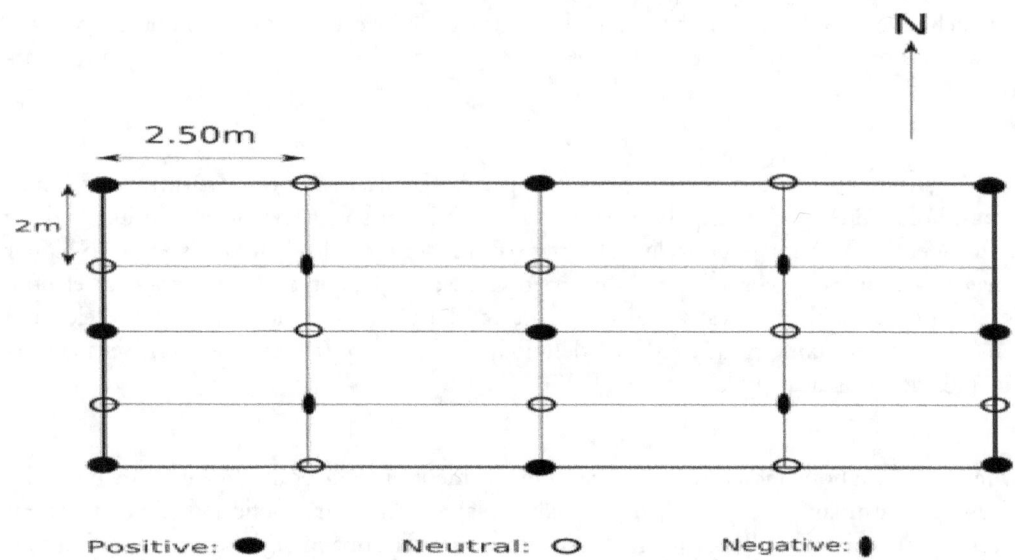

The Hartmann Grid

Source: http://www.lysator.liu.se/~rasmus/skepticism/dowsing.html

Why I mention this here is because Doctor Hartmann has conducted a lot of medical research relating to Hartmann lines and he claims all cases of cancer can be related to these lines !

Curry lines, on the other hand, have been discovered by Swiss physician Manfred Curry in 1950s, they also form a grid of 3.5m by 3.5m, are 40cm wide and stretch in direction of northwest-southeast and northeast-southwest. They are also perpendicular to each other and also cross previously mentioned Hartmman lines at 45 degrees angle.

So Curry lines are further apart (3.5m) than Hartman (2m) are wider (40cm as opposed to 21cm) and cross Hartmann lines at 45 degrees angle. Jointly they form rather dense network of radiation with many pathogenic crosses. Both are as shown in next picture.

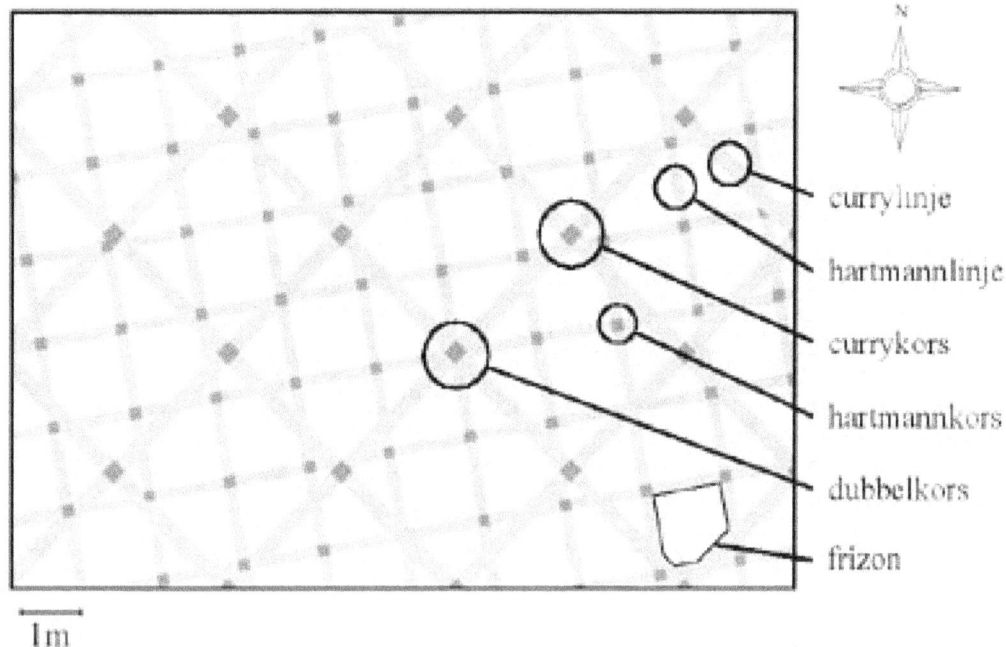

currylinje

hartmannlinje

currykors

hartmannkors

dubbelkors

frizon

1 m

Source: http://www.lysator.liu.se/~rasmus/skepticism/dowsing.html

How to find the lines

Hartmann

Finding these lines is not hard at all. But it requires unconventional method known as dowsing. And no, it's not magic nor does anything to do with it. Important thing is that no other "scientific" method will easily find Hartman and Curry lines. Dowsing is not something magicians use, it's the real thing which I easily and quite successfully applied in my flat and countryside house. Dowsing rods respond to magnetic forces and work better if paired. The important thing is that you hold them loosely in your hands pointing forward in parallel and perpendicular to forces (lines) you are trying to detect. When you cross perpendicular line they will simply close in to one another. If you want to find N-S (S-N) Hartmann line you have to walk W-E (or E-W doesn't matter) and if you want to find W-E line (E-W) you have to walk N-S (or S-N doesn't matter). At one point rods will turn perpendicularly to your direction with quite some force ! Simple as that ! Imagine the force necessary to pull the rods ? No magic, pure physics. If you want more training check videos on Youtube or similar services.

Typical dowsing rods:

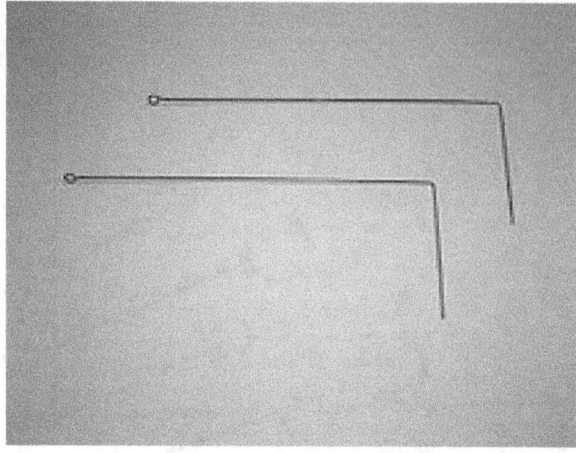

Source: http://en.wikipedia.org/wiki/Dowsing

More detailed procedure to find the lines goes like this:

1. Take 2 pieces of wire 40cm long.

2. Bent each piece in 1/3 of length perpendicularly so you can hold shorter part nicely.

3. Use compass to locate N-S direction as we will be looking for E-W lines

4. Walk by each wall in your house holding dowsing rods loosely in your hands pointing them north. So walk by wall as it is but point rods north ! You will see that every 2.5m or so rods will automatically point east-west meaning you found latitude lines. The important thing is to hold rods loosely so they may sway easily and to point them north all the time! Using this method cover room by room and wall by wall one at the time and point the dot on the wall where you found the line. Also mark that line on wall as N-S line so you know where it crosses the wall.

5. Now again slowly walk by all walls again but pointing rods east-west and again you will see they will turn N-S again every 2m or so. Again mark dot on wall so you know where lines are and describe it E-W.

6. When you finish all rooms you can measure with meter all walls, detected dots and draw a sketch of layout of your flat/house or better still use original design of house and only mark dots you detected. Make sure to correctly indicate where you found particular type of dots   N-S, E-W dots.

7. If done correctly you can easily draw straight lines through all N-S dots on layout/scheme in all rooms and convince yourself these lines really exist! Right in your house! And you or your children may be sleeping on them! For years! God forbid should you sleep on crossings…

Similar thing is with Curry lines. But your rods must be pointed northwest-southeast direction to find northeast-southwest lines and vice-versa. You will probably find lots of lines by walls but judging by size and angle of lines pulling the rods (21cm for Hartmann and 40cm for Curry; Curry lines cross Hartmann lines at 45% angle, look at above diagram) you can make out which are which with a bit of effort. And the effort is well worth it.

Not only did I change my bed at home according to layout of flat but also working desk at work as I was sitting right on N-E line Hartmann line for 2 years! Remember Hartmann lines form grid around 2m by 2.5m and are 21cm wide, while Curry lines are much wider and form grid being 3.5m by 3.5m apart and 40cm wide.

Infectious Agents

Worldwide, an estimated 17.8% of neoplasms are associated with infections; this percentage ranges from less than 10% in high-income countries to 25% in African countries[22]. Viruses account for most infection-caused cancers. Viruses are the usual infectious agents that cause cancer.

Human papillomavirus, Epstein Barr virus, Kaposi's sarcoma-associated herpes virus, human T-lymphotropic virus 1, HIV, HBV, and HCV are associated with risks for cervical cancer, anogenital cancer, skin cancer, nasopharyngeal cancer, Burkitt's lymphoma, Hodgkin's lymphoma, Kaposi's sarcoma, adult T-cell leukemia, B-cell lymphoma, and liver cancer. Human papillomavirus is directly mutagenic by inducing the viral genes E6 and E7, whereas HBV is believed to be indirectly mutagenic by generating reactive oxygen species through chronic inflammation. Human T-lymphotropic virus is directly mutagenic, whereas HCV (like HBV) is believed to produce oxidative stress in infected cells and thus to act indirectly through chronic inflammation. Infection-related inflammation is the major risk factor for cancer, and almost all viruses linked to cancer have been shown to activate the inflammatory marker, NF-κB[23].

What does this mean and what should I do ?

In this chapter we roughly summarized types of radiation and touched upon virus infections as external hazard. We pointed out radiation that can be linked directly to cancer such as ionizing radiation. There can be silent killers as well like usual electromagnetic radiation which exceeds given threshold values. If you live near high-voltage power rails or above underground train or similar things you are strongly advised to obtain measurements electromagnetic radiation in your living place. Maybe even more importantly perform analysis of Hartman and Curry lines in your house. It costs only 2 pieces of 40cm long wire and a bit of effort. And some won't be laughing when they found them in bedroom.

Some cancers are related to virus infections. And any sort of permanent inflammation is not good. For example permanent stomach inflammation can lead to ulcer and cancer. For volatile viruses like papillomavirus the obvious thing is to protect yourself from contraction.

---

[22] P.Pisani, d.M. Parkin, J. Ferlay, Cancer and infection. Cancer epidemiol. Biomarkers Prev.6 387-400(1997;

[23] Y. S. Guan, Q. He, M. Q. Wang, and P. Li. Nuclear factor kappa B and hepatitis viruses. Expert Opin. Ther. Targets. 12:265–280 (2008)

2. Something called pH

pH Value

Acidic and alkaline are two extremes that describe a chemical property of chemicals. Mixing acids and alkaline can cancel out or neutralize their extreme effects. A substance that is neither acidic nor basic is neutral. The pH scale measures how acidic or alkaline a substance is. The pH scale ranges from 0 to 14. A pH of 7 is neutral. A pH less than 7 is acidic. A pH greater than 7 is alkaline.

The pH scale is logarithmic and as a result, each whole pH value below 7 is ten times more acidic than the next higher value. For example, pH 4 is ten times more acidic than pH 5 and 100 times (10 times 10) more acidic than pH 6. The same holds true for pH values above 7, each of which is ten times more alkaline than the next lower whole value. For example, pH 10 is ten times more alkaline than pH 9 and 100 times (10 times 10) more alkaline than pH 8. Ideal pH for blood is 7.4.[24]

Water molecules exist in equilibrium with hydrogen ions and hydroxide ions. Ions are atoms with deficite or excess of electrons and are therefore positively or negatively charged.

$H2O <--> H+ + OH-$

H+ is positively charged meaning it lacks one electron and OH- is negatively charged meaning it has excess of one electron. The pH scale, (0 - 14) indicate the concentration of H+ and OH-ions in solution.

BOTH H+ and OH- ions are always present in any solution. A solution is acidic if the H+ are in excess. A solution is alkaline, if the OH- ions are in excess. Therefore acidic food is negatively charged and body tends to neutralize this by either:

-   filter out H+ ions out as urine
-   storing acid away in fatty cells
-   neutralize it's charge with calcium from bones

The following diagram gives some relationships which summarizes the issue:

[24] http://www.elmhurst.edu/

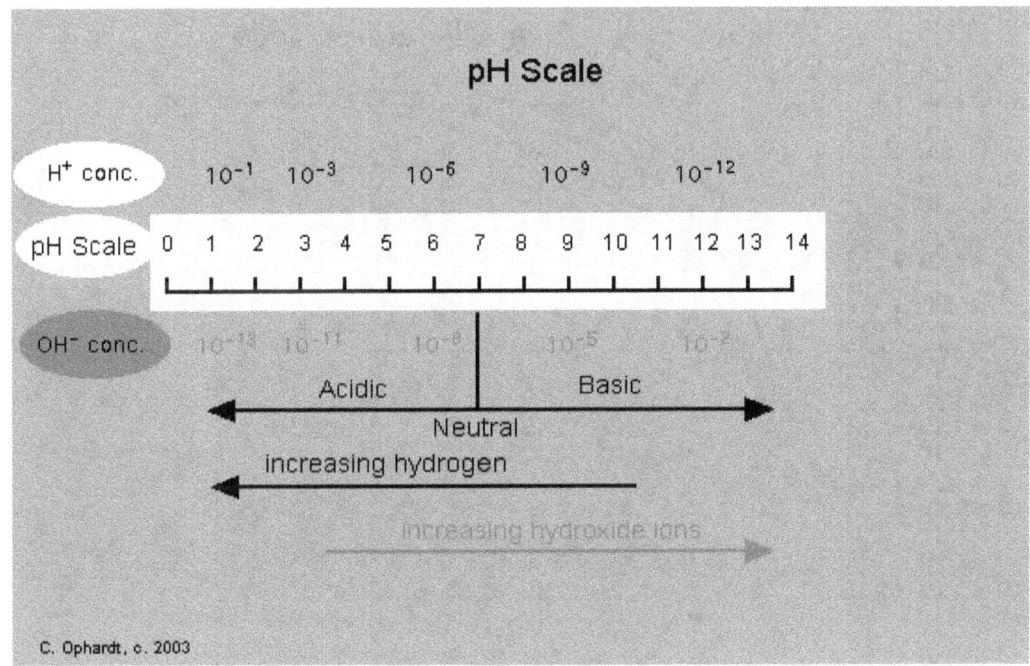

Source: http://www.elmhurst.edu/

Effect of pH on the oxygen supply

As blood returns to the lung, carbon dioxide dissociates from hemoglobin and enters the alveoli. This process is associated with a reduction in blood PCO_2 with an attendant decrease in $[H^+]$ due to the decrease in blood carbonic acid. As can be seen from following diagram, pH value affects ability of blood to carry and supply cells with oxygen.

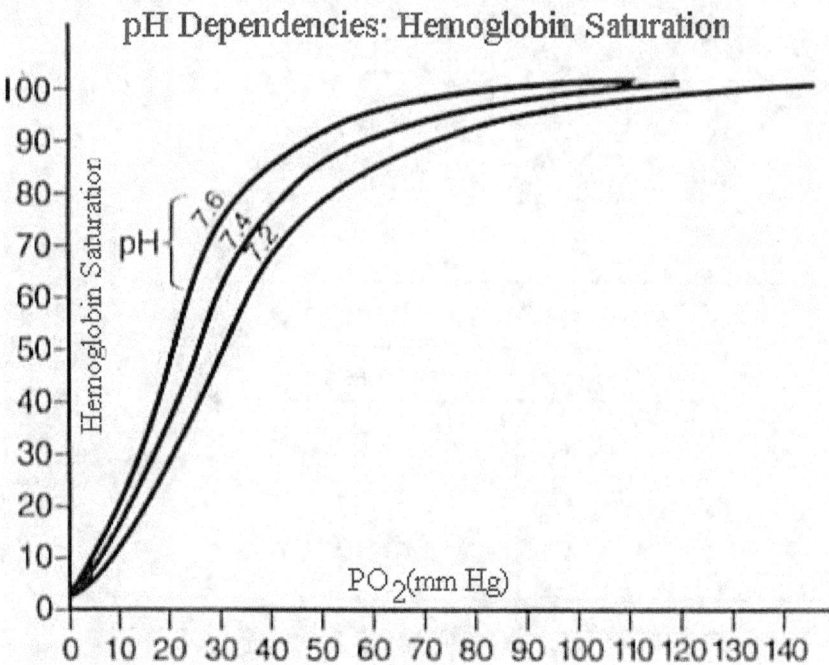

pH Dependencies: Hemoglobin Saturation

Source: http://www.anesthesia2000.com/physics/Chemistry_Physics/physics21.htm

A leftward and upward shift, if we examine the curve results in a higher degree of hemoglobin saturation and any given oxygen tension. This increased saturation creates conditions favoring oxygen transport to the tissues.

The tissue, as a result of metabolism, is producing carbon dioxide and therefore the blood, now at the capillary level, is exposed to higher levels of carbon dioxide (increasing blood carbonic acid in decreasing pH). This condition causes a shift to the right in the hemoglobin-oxygen saturation curve which means that there will be reduced hemoglobin saturation in any given oxygen partial pressure. Reduced hemoglobin saturation means that more oxygen has dissociated at that particular partial pressure we chose, thus making more oxygen molecules available to the tissue[25].

Optimal pH for saliva is 6.4 to 6.8. A reading lower than 6.4 is indicative of insufficient alkaline reserves. After eating, the saliva pH should rise to 7.8 or higher. Unless this occurs, the body has alkaline mineral deficiencies (mainly calcium and magnesium) and will not assimilate food very well. To deviate from ideal salivary pH for an extended time invites illness.

Urinary pH Test: The pH of the urine indicates how the body is working to maintain the proper pH of the blood. The pH of urine indicates the effectiveness of the body to regulate pH via the kidneys, adrenals, lungs and gonads through the buffer salts and hormones. Urine can provide a

---

[25] http://www.anesthesia2000.com/physics/Chemistry_Physics/physics21.htm

fairly accurate picture of body chemistry, because the kidneys filter out the buffer salts of pH regulation and provide values based on what the body is eliminating. Urine pH can vary from around 4.5 to 9.0 for its extremes, but the ideal range is 5.8 to 6.8.

Breakdown of glucose produces acid

CO_2 and $H+$ are produced during the breakdown of glucose, and are removed from the muscle via the blood. The production and removal of CO_2 and $H+$, together with the use and transport of oxygen, cause chemical changes in the blood. These chemical changes, unless offset by other physiological functions, cause the pH of the blood to drop. If the pH of the body gets too low (below 7), a condition known as acidosis results. This can be very serious, because many of the chemical reactions that occur in the body, especially those involving proteins, are pH-dependent. Ideally, the pH of the blood should be maintained at 7.4.

During exercise, the muscles use up oxygen as they convert chemical energy in glucose to mechanical energy. Formula is as follows $C6H12O6 + 6O2 + 6H2O \rightarrow 12H2O + 6\ CO2$. This O2 comes from hemoglobin in the blood. CO_2 and $H+$ are produced during the breakdown of glucose, and are removed from the muscle via the blood. Therefore breakdown of glucose directly acidifies your body. And caner likes acidic bodies.

Dr. Warburg's was rewarded Nobel Prize for discovering that cells fundamentally turn cancerous when their mitochondria (the energy factory of the cell) becomes damaged. Usually this damage results from lack of oxygen or caused by toxins. Once the mitochondria have been damaged, the cell principally produces energy without oxygen by fermenting glucose or sugar. Cancer cell fermentation is like lactic acid fermentation with following formula:

$$C_6H_{12}O_6 \rightarrow 2\ CH_3CHOHCOOH$$

Cancer cells have 15 times more insulin receptors than normal cells. The insulin dose helps to target chemotherapy into cancer cells because they have so many more insulin receptors. Oxygen and ozone treatment - the key to this therapy is getting elevated concentrations of oxygen into the body or tumor using various means. Dr. Otto Warburg showed that cancer cells do not occur in a healthy, oxygenated environment. Many think lack of oxygen is the prime cause of all cancers. An impressive variety of new ways to introduce oxygen into the body are emerging including pressure chambers, liquid oxygen, peroxide, chemical compounds, acid/alkaline balancing, injections, and ozone treatments. Flooding cells with oxygen may retard the growth of cancer cells or even help to return them to normal. From here came idea of ozonated water or water with 2 oxygen atoms (instead of one).

"Deprive a cell 60% of its oxygen and it will turn cancerous. Deprive a cell 35% of its oxygen for 48 hours and it may become cancerous". - Dr. Otto Warburg.

Here is the perfect place to quote relation of cancer with cell specialized functions from
http://www.healingcancernaturally.com/warburgcancer-cause-prevention.html

"The early history of life on our planet indicates that life existed on earth before the earth's atmosphere contained free oxygen gas. The living cells must therefore have been fermenting cells then, and, as fossils show, they were undifferentiated single cells. Only when free oxygen appeared in the atmosphere - some billion years ago - did the higher development of life set in, to produce the plant and animal kingdoms from the fermenting, undifferentiated single cells. What the philosophers of life have called "Evolution créatrice" has been and is therefore the work of oxygen.

The reverse process, the dedifferentiation of life, takes place today in greatest amount before our eyes in cancer development, which is another expression for dedifferentiation. To be sure, cancer development takes place even in the presence of free oxygen gas in the atmosphere, but this oxygen may not penetrate in sufficient quantity into the growing body cells, or the respiratory apo-enzymes of the growing body cells may not be saturated with the active groups. In any case, during the cancer development the oxygen-respiration always falls, fermentation appears, and the highly differentiated cells are transformed to fermenting anaerobes, which have lost all their body functions and retain only the now useless property of growth. Thus, when respiration disappears, life does not disappear, but the meaning of life disappears, and what remains are growing machines that destroy the body in which they grow".

What does this mean and what should I do ?

It means pH and oxygen are very important ! And there is much you can do. First test your pH of saliva to evaluate how acidic your body is as indicator of what is your risk of developing cancer. pH will be detailed in next chapter on food as well but it is important to avoid lifestyle which includes oxygen deficient scenarios (particular occupations, habitats…) and reduce intake of sugar (glucose).

As oxygen part is concerned you can do much to improve you chances with no cost at all:

1. Fresh air. Increase the amount of oxygen in the air you breathe by allowing fresh air into every room of your home, office and transportation

2. Deep breathing. Improper breathing causes oxygen deficiency. Use the full capacity of your lungs by expanding both the chest and lower abdomen. Practice deep breathing for a few minutes every day. If you feel depressed, try breathing more deeply. Deep breathing also contributes to moving the lymph.

3. Aerobic exercise increases the capacity of the heart to pump blood and increases the capacity of the lungs.

4. Eat smaller nutrient-dense meals (no empty-calorie junk food). Overeating causes oxygen deficiency. Do you feel tired after a big meal? Vitamin F increases the oxygen carrying capacity of the hemoglobin in red blood cells. Eat an alkaline diet and create an alkaline condition in the body.

5. Avoid carbon monoxide (vehicle exhaust, fumes from gas stoves & heaters) that reduces the oxygen carrying capacity of the blood.

6. Drink ozonated water.

3. Food consumption

Food and tobacco usually classify as number one cause of cancers. Everybody knows alcohol is bad but people usually oversee the fact that junk food, although tasteful is the silent killer. We should therefore refer back shortly to chapter about cell growth. Junk food will not make your cells grow and duplicate in normal way and malignant processes are just question of time. Junk food also inhibits your immune system and reduces oxygen supply to cells in the long run. Normal cell growth and duplication requires nutrients which you will not find in most processed food civilized people consume today. Herby it is worth knowing two facts:

One is that food processed using pasteurization or other thermal methods (frying, cooking) looses most of it's nutritional value and you basically consume "junk" your body does not need. Now imagine what are consequences of filling your body with junk for years ?

Second is that highly processed food like salami, candies and can food is also not advisable because it contains various additives ranging from nitrates to antibiotics, and from aspartame to saccharine. When digested these are broken up to toxic and poisonous substances.

Here it must be mentioned that sticky, gluey food without fibers sticks to membrane of your colon and just rots there. Norman Walker wrote about this at lengths. And it can easily be connected to various chronic diseases including excessive pressure on heart from gas buildup. Grown up people have few pounds of this rotting garbage inside themselves which is major factory of disease and some even develop what is called "leaky gut" syndrome. This means toxins penetrate colon wall and enter blood stream and it is than up to liver to clean them up. Liver is only able to do this to an extent and malfunctions after some time. Than it is kidneys turn to feel the heat etc. So healthy colon is number 1. precondition for at least two things:

a) normal absorption of nutrients needed for proper functioning of cell growth and energy supply

b) healthy body with healthy blood and healthy internal organs

To elaborate a bit let's see what food we consume:

- proteins
- carbohydrates
- fats
- minerals and vitamins etc.

These ingredients are mixed up in variety of food stuffs like:

- animal meat, fish

- sugar derivatives

- breadstuff

- milk, diary products

- fruits and vegetables

Animal meat (proteins)

Proteins are important part of human cells and tissues. Proteins are composed of simpler parts called amino-acids. Amino acids are divided in essential and non-essential (meaning human body can synthesize non-essential ones). Humans today get most proteins from animal meat. When we digest animal meat or animal proteins they have to be broken up first by enzymes to amino acids and than "reassembled" again as human proteins. This requires lot of energy, stresses our digestion system and that is why we are more tired after big meat meal than before it. On average westerners consume at least three times more animal meat than is necessary for average occupation. So think about that, three times more than is necessary to sustain average person.

When consuming animal proteins we really need to look at what actually we are consuming. Today's cows, pigs, chickens don't live in natural environment, they don't feed naturally and are stuffed to their necks with antibiotics, growth hormones, steroids and other baddies served by meat industry. Their food is usually full of pesticides. On top of that before being slaughtered and during slaughter animals are "brutalized" and they produce lots of adrenalin that is being pumped into their blood and absorbed in their meat. Worst of all may be poultry meat where chickens, turkeys are during cleansing process drowned for hours in water containing their excrements before being packed up to supermarket and served as delicious meal. That's why "organic" food is picking up in Europe as a hit. Of course it usually cost 30%-75% more but it is obviously worth it. When USA will join this trend it remains to be seen.

Antibiotics, growth hormones, and adrenalin in this tasty meat doesn't go away with cooking and frying. No, they stay there beside other innutritious elements do be consumed by – you dear reader ! And filling body with this "junk" or toxic stuff will have consequences. Let me say that again – will have consequences sooner or later. It is destined to have consequences. As people grow old their resistance to diseases and malignant processes (older people produce less enzymes, they build up stocks of toxic byproducts of incomplete digestion, chronically lack necessary nutrients for cell growth and are overall disabled to expel all junk that accumulated over the years) increases significantly as well as their risk of getting cancer in digestion system or somewhere else.

Frying or cooking animal meat also destroys much of nutritional value, if there was any in the first place. Byproducts of animal protein digestion are nitrogen which ultimately contributes to corresponding formation of uric acid. Elevated levels of uric acid, especially if associated with other diseases, can begin to precipitate into crystals and cause gout.

Carbohydrates

Popular myth exists that ever since Egyptians sawn wheat to feed the nation it is essential to human growth. It is also true that too much carbohydrates (bread, beer, pasta…) causes obesity. During digestion carbohydrates are in the end broken down to complex (polysaccharides, disaccharides), and simple sugars (monosaccharide). Simple sugar in the form of glucose and fructose are at the end of digestion absorbed in the blood stream to be used for energy. Liver regulates level of glucose in blood. Excess glucose is converted in the liver to glycogen by hormone insulin. And why cancer loves glucose and insulin is written in next sub-chapter.

Aside from likely cancer related problems, consuming too much carbohydrates can lead to diabetes messing up your insulin production and glucose level. National Health and Nutrition Examination Survey found obesity is better linked with increased sugar intake than consumption of fat[26].

Sugar problems

During evolution process sugar was never eaten by Neanderthals or homo sapiens in it's industrial disaccharide form. And evolution and genetics went fine without it meaning it's totally useless in our digestion or better to say we did not develop any special need for it and therefore it is redundant. It is known fact that table sugar (sucrose) and other sugars lead to diabetes. It is less known fact that sugar:

a) feeds cancer cells disproportional more than normal cells

b) ultimately lowers your pH and makes your body acidic as result of glucose transformation

   to energy (creation of H+ ions)

c) reduces blood capacity to deliver oxygen because of lower pH

d) inhibits your immune system via influence on neutrophil leukocytes

e) inhibits vitamin C intake as uses the same receptors as glucose to enter the cell membrane

f) also inhibits „autophagy process" described earlier, where damaged and worn out

   mitochondria is recycled

That's six for price of one. Indeed a worthy product if you think about it.

Here it is worth remembering that Dr. Warburg's discovered that cells fundamentally turn cancerous when their mitochondria (the energy factory of the cell) becomes damaged. Usually this damage results from lack of oxygen caused by toxins, or by lack of CoQ10 - crucial enzyme in energy production in the cell. Once the mitochondrial enzymes have been damaged, the cell principally produces energy without oxygen by fermenting glucose or sugar.

Cancer cells have 15 times more insulin receptors than normal cells. The insulin dose helps to target chemotherapy into cancer cells because they have so many more insulin receptors.

Readers will recognize insulin as being the hormone used to treat diabetes. Secreted by the pancreas in healthy people, insulin is a powerful hormone with many actions in the human body, a principal one being to manage the delivery of glucose across cell membranes into cells. Insulin communicates its messages to cells by joining up with specific insulin receptors scattered on the outer surface of the cell membranes. Having much more insulin receptors than normal cells means that the effect of administered insulin will be much greater on cancer cells than on normal cells.

---

[26] http://www.cdc.gov/nchs/nhanes.htm

It is a well-known scientific fact that cancer cells have a voracious appetite for glucose. Glucose is their unique source of energy, and because of the relatively inefficient way cancer cells burn this fuel, they use up a great deal of it. This is one reason why cancer patients lose so much weight. Because cancer cells require so much glucose, they virtually steal it away from the body's normal cells, thus starving them.

The interesting connection between cancer cells and insulin is that recent findings published in the scientific medical literature report that cancer cells actually manufacture and secrete their own insulin.

Animal models have shown that increasing sucrose intake increases the neurotransmitter serotonin, important for mood balancing, suggesting that eating sugar can make us feel better when depressed[27]. Although consuming sugar may result in enhanced mood, anyone who experiences this "sugar high" must pay a steep price. This is because numerous studies have shown that increased sugar intake dramatically decreases the immune response.

Short-term hyperglycemia (elevated blood sugar) affects all major components of innate immunity and impairs the ability of the individual to fight infection[28]. The white blood cells are the primary mediators of the immune response. Neutrophils are a type of white blood cell that act as an important first-line-of-defense in the immune system by engulfing (phagocytizing) pathogens. Hyperglycemia has been shown to decrease neutrophil activity in numerous studies[29]. One study showed that increased glucose levels decreased neutrophils' ability to engulf several pathogens such as Staphylococcus epidermidis, Staphylococcus aureus, and Escherichia coli[30]. A similar study showed that poor blood sugar control in diabetic patients decreased neutrophil activity against Klebsiella pneumoniae[31]. Specifically, neutrophils experienced a decrease in their movement and their ability to engulf and kill pathogens, an increase in leukocyte apoptosis (programmed cell death), and a reduction in lymph node retention capacity. Additionally, lowering of blood glucose has been shown to significantly improve neutrophil activity.

There is something called a "phagocytic index" which tells you how rapidly a particular macrophage or lymphocyte can gobble up a virus, bacteria, or cancer cell.

We know that glucose and vitamin C have similar chemical structures, so what happens when the sugar levels go up? They compete with one another upon entering the cells via insulin-mediated tunneling mechanism. And the thing that mediates the entry of glucose into the cells is the same thing that mediates the entry of vitamin C into the cells. If there is more glucose around, there is going to be less vitamin C allowed into the cell. Both molecules require

[27] Smolders I, Loo JV, Sarre S, et al. Effects of dietary sucrose on hippocampal serotonin release: a microdialysis study in the freely-moving rat. Br J Nutr. 2001 Aug

[28] Turina M, Fry DE, Polk HC Jr. Acute hyperglycemia and the innate immune system; Crit Care Med. 2005 Jul

[29] Patel KL. Impact of tight glucose control on postoperative infection rates and wound healing in cardiac surgery patients.

[30] Van Oss CJ. Influence of glucose levels on the in vitro phagocytosis of bacteria by human neutrophils. Infect Immun. 1971 Jul

[31] Lin JC, Siu LK, Fung CP, et al. Impaired phagocytosis of capsular serotypes K1 or K2 Klebsiella pneumoniae in type 2 diabetes mellitus patients with poor glycemic control. J Clin Endocrinol Metab. 2006 Aug

help from the pancreatic hormone insulin before they can penetrate cell membranes using special "pumps." White blood cells have more insulin pumps and they may contain 20 times the amount of vitamin C as ordinary cells. It doesn't take much: a blood sugar value of 120 mg/dl (6 mmol/L) reduces the phagocytic index by 75%. Phagocytic index tells us how quickly bacteria are removed from our body. So when you eat sugar, think of your immune system slowing down to a crawl[32].

In the last 20 years, the sugar consumption of the average North American has increased from 26 to 135 lbs of sugar per person per year. Prior to 1900 (when cardiovascular disease and cancer was virtually unknown) average consumption was only 5 lbs per person per year. That figure correlates nicely with increased number of cancer cases.

Here we are getting a little bit closer to the roots of disease. It doesn't matter what disease we are talking about, whether we are talking about a common cold or about cardiovascular disease, or cancer or osteoporosis, the root is always going to be at the cellular and molecular level, and more often than not insulin is going to have its hand in it, if not totally controlling it.

The health dangers which ingesting sugar on habitual basis creates are certain. Simple sugars have been observed to aggravate asthma, move mood swings, provoke personality changes, muster mental illness, nourish nervous disorders, deliver diabetes, hurry heart disease, grow gallstones, hasten hypertension, and add arthritis[33].

Replacement for sugar

Stevia, pure and simple. It contains no calories and is 30 times more sweet than sugar – meaning you have to use 30 times smaller dose. It's replacement for aspartame as well. Japan forced Coca-cola to use stevia in it's products for Japanese market but western countries did not think of that.

Vegetables, fruit

Vegetables and fruit are extremely good for human body. Not least because they are rich in minerals and vitamins. They also contain fibers which are necessary to clean and regulate proper bowel movement. They are also usually alkaline food rich in antioxidants like broccoli meaning they reduce impact of free radicals. Needles to say one should consume fruits and vegetables that was not treated with pesticides and alike as not to digest harmful toxins. Unfortunately much of beneficial elements in vegetables are destroyed in thermal treatment like cooking. But beware vitamin C is destroyed with heat over 70 degrees and it leaks out into the cooking water because it is a water soluble vitamin.

---

[32] http://www.healingdaily.com/detoxification-diet/sugar.htm

[33] http://www.healingdaily.com/detoxification-diet/sugar.htm

Alkaline, acid foodstuffs

Alkaline and acidity were described in corresponding chapter. To repeat here, pH value means "Potential of Hydrogen" and vary between 0 (most acid) and 14 (most alkaline). Healthy limit for human body is between 7 - 7.5

In introduction we mentioned that cancer does not like alkaline and sugarless environment. On the opposite it does like acid and sugary environment. So one really crucial element in fight against cancer is that we eat alkaline food and avoid acid and candies or other sugar related products. Therefore it is absolutely necessary to test pH value of your body. You can do this by commercially available ph tests for saliva and urine. It is most desirable that your pH value is above 7. Sodium bicarbonate is powerful alkaline drink. And that is a fact. There are numerous cases where people diagnosed with cancer pointed out sodium bicarbonate as most effective weapon. There is also enough evidence where Italian doctor Simoncini (oncologist) is treating patients with soda solution infusions that suggest great success even in cases crossed out by official medicine. According to him sodium bicarbonate destroys *Candida albicans* - yeast that causes cancer.

Few examples of alkaline food:

ALKALIZING FOODS		
VEGETABLES	FRUITS	OTHER
Garlic	Apple	Apple Cider Vinegar
Asparagus	Apricot	Bee Pollen
Fermented Veggies	Avocado	Lecithin Granules
Watercress	Banana (high glycemic)	Probiotic Cultures
Beets	Cantaloupe	Green Juices
Broccoli	Cherries	Veggies Juices
Brussel sprouts	Currants	Fresh Fruit Juice
Cabbage	Dates/Figs	Organic Milk
Carrot	Grapes	(unpasteurized)
Cauliflower	Grapefruit	Mineral Water
Celery	Lime	Alkaline Antioxidant Water
Chard	Honeydew Melon	Green Tea
Chlorella	Nectarine	Herbal Tea
Collard Greens	Orange	Dandelion Tea
Cucumber	Lemon	Ginseng Tea
Eggplant	Peach	Banchi Tea
Kale	Pear	Kombucha
Kohlrabi	Pineapple	
Lettuce	All Berries	SWEETENERS
Mushrooms	Tangerine	Stevia
Mustard Greens	Tomato	
Dulce	Tropical Fruits	SPICES/SEASONINGS
Dandelions	Watermelon	Cinnamon
Edible Flowers		Curry

Onions	PROTEIN	Ginger
Parsnips (high glycemic)	Eggs	Mustard
Peas	Whey Protein Powder	Chili Pepper
Peppers	Cottage Cheese	Sea Salt
Pumpkin	Chicken Breast	Miso
Rutabaga	Yogurt	Tamari
Sea Veggies	Almonds	All Herbs
Spirulina	Chestnuts	
Sprouts	Tofu (fermented)	ORIENTAL VEGETABLES
Squashes	Flax Seeds	Maitake
Alfalfa	Pumpkin Seeds	Daikon
Barley Grass	Tempeh (fermented)	Dandelion Root
Wheat Grass	Squash Seeds	Shitake
Wild Greens	Sunflower Seeds	Kombu
Nightshade Veggies	Millet	Reishi
	Sprouted Seeds	Nori
	Nuts	Umeboshi
		Wakame
		Sea Veggies

Few examples of acid food:

FATS & OILS	NUTS & BUTTERS	DRUGS & CHEMICALS
Avocado Oil	Cashews	Chemicals
Canola Oil	Brazil Nuts	Drugs, Medicinal
Corn Oil	Peanuts	Drugs, Psychedelic
Hemp Seed Oil	Peanut Butter	Pesticides
Flax Oil	Pecans	Herbicides
Lard	Tahini	
Olive Oil	Walnuts	ALCOHOL
Safflower Oil		Beer
Sesame Oil	ANIMAL PROTEIN	Spirits
Sunflower Oil	Beef	Hard Liquor
	Carp	Wine
FRUITS	Clams	
Cranberries	Fish	BEANS & LEGUMES
	Lamb	Black Beans
GRAINS	Lobster	Chick Peas
Rice Cakes	Mussels	Green Peas
Wheat Cakes	Oyster	Kidney Beans
Amaranth	Pork	Lentils
Barley	Rabbit	Lima Beans
Buckwheat	Salmon	Pinto Beans
Corn	Shrimp	Red Beans
Oats (rolled)	Scallops	Soy Beans
Quinoi	Tuna	Soy Milk
Rice (all)	Turkey	White Beans

Rye	Venison	Rice Milk
Spelt		Almond Milk
Kamut	PASTA (WHITE)	
Wheat	Noodles	
Hemp Seed Flour	Macaroni	
	Spaghetti	
DAIRY		
Cheese, Cow	OTHER	
Cheese, Goat	Distilled Vinegar	
Cheese, Processed	Wheat Germ	
Cheese, Sheep	Potatoes	
Milk		
Butter		

It can't be stressed enough how important it is to avoid acid food and that relates to drinks as well. It's safest to avoid almost all types of refined beverages like colas, soda, even juice from your local store as it is usually low concentration, highly processed juice with lots of added sugar and with little nutritional value.

Importance of fresh juice

There are few things as good for human body as freshly squeezed juice. It can be from all kind of vegetables and fruits. People should drink only drink juice from fresh vegetables or fruit. And fresh juice oxidizes very quickly in fresh air so you must drink it within 15 min if possible and than imagine what quality is juice that sits in stores for few months ?

In fact fresh juice should be your main source of nutrients. Organic grown vegetables is not stuffed with hormones or antibiotics or adrenalin and contains all kind of nutrients in extreme quantities that human body can use immediately without any load on your digestive tract. Here we must mention the work of Walker Norman who originally started to practice diet with vegetable juice, had tremendous success and lived … 113 years ! For more on crucial importance of fresh juice on human health I definitely recommend his books on salads and juices.

Drinking lots of fresh juice from carrot, red beet, apple etc. (even liter per day) is excellent preventive measure as your cells are than provided with enough healthy nutrients for their growth and division minimizing the chance of malignant processes to occur. It is equally good for people that already have cancer diagnosed, especially with combination of bowels cleaning.

But you must be cautious how juice is prepared. It should not be prepared in high speed blenders which warm the juice up because heat kills nutrients remember ? It should be prepared in low rotating juicers, which act like hydraulic presses and squeeze juice out by sheer force without heat. Juicer "Oscar 1000" is a nice example of high quality juicer.

Milk and dairy products

It is usually thought that milk and dairy products are good for everybody. Think again. Cow milk is rich in casein which is used extensively in glue industry and which in digestion leaves lots of slime behind which serves as breeding place for bacteria. Lots of decomposing bacteria are not good for health.

After all cow milk is intended for calf of few hundred kilos not humans who are several times lighter. Best deary product is goat milk if you can obtain it in fresh state. It has 3 times as little casein than cow milk and much better for you. Stuff like yogurt it somewhat better especially kefir like products enriched with digestion friendly bacteria.

Conventional milk (and meat) products are very likely to contain antibiotics which harm and destroy the good (beneficial) intestinal flora This apparently both impedes proper digestion/optimal mineral nutrient assimilation and immune system performance and contributes to sporadic Candidiasis epidemic (Candidiasis being defined as "overgrowth in the gastrointestinal tract of the usually benign yeast [or fungus] Candida albicans"). Candida fungus overgrowth has become widespread apparently due to indiscriminate antibiotics use in the food chain.

Yeast infection

Nice way to test yourself for yeast infection is to spit in glass of water in the morning when you wake up. If after 30 min there are visible strings (like hydra legs) going from top to bottom of glass...you are suffering from yeast infection. And that can lead to many diseases, contributing to cancer as well. If that is the case avoid food in which yeast shoes up meaning milk, cheese, yogurt, bread etc.

Chlorine

"Chlorine is pesticide"[34]. As defined by US Environment protection Agency. And you drink it. A lot. It was also used as chemical weapon in WW1. Chlorine combines with other natural compounds to form cancerogenous proven trihalomethanes[35] (chlorination byproducts), or THMs one of which is chloroform. These chlorine by-products trigger the production of free radicals in the body, causing cell damage, and are highly carcinogenic. Chlorine is also suspected to contribute to hardening of the arteries, the primary cause of heart disease. Even a WHO report on chlorine admits that "An increased risk of bladder cancer appears to be associated with the consumption of chlorinated tap water in a population-based, case–control study of adults consuming chlorinated or non-chlorinated water for half of their lifetimes"[36].

Recent study led by Manolis Kogevinas and published in magazine Environmental Health Perspectives revealed that people who had swim in chlorine treated swimming pools in Barcelona showed large rise in markers of DNA damage that can lead to cancer.

---

[34] http://www.epa.gov/kidshometour/products/bleach.htm

[35] Drinking water criteria document on Trihalomethanes; US Environment Protection Agency, 1994

[36] http://www.who.int/water_sanitation_health/dwq/chlorine.pdf

This view is backed up by other medical professionals. So for example Dr. J.M. Price states that "Cancer risks among people drinking chlorinated water is 93% higher than among those whose water does not contain chlorine." Dr. Riddle, Ph.D. has stated, "Each day in America, about 30 cases of rectal cancer may be associated with THMs (chlorination by-products) in drinking water." Dr. Robert Carlson from University of Minesota claims that "chlorine is the greatest crippler and killer of modern times".

Current limit for chlorine in water as set by Environment Protection Agency is 4mg/L. Limit for all trihalomethanes combined (Bromoform, Chloroform, Bromodichloromethane, Dibromochloromethane) is 0.08mg/L. You can test levels of chlorine in your water supply via various testers.

So what to do ? At your house you can install water filters which filter chlorine alongside others toxic chemicals. You should most certainly install shower filters as well because chlorine easily evaporates and showers are perfect place to inhale lots of chlorine. Better filters utilize something called reverse osmosis to filter out practically everything aside water molecules. But water that lost most minerals is also not healthy in long run and as such should be remineralized before consumption.

Tobacco

So much has been said on tobacco it makes little point of elaborating the point. It contains 40+ cancerogenous elements and majority of lung cancer are caused by tobacco smokers. And it is more addictive than heroin as average time to get off is 2 years.

Aspartame&artificial sweeteners

Aspartame is artificial sweetener which can be found in wide range of products from chewing gums to soda drinks. Practically anything that says "sugar free" is likely to contain aspartame. Upon ingestion, aspartame breaks down into natural residual components, including aspartic acid, phenylalanine, methanol, and further breakdown products including formaldehyde and formic acid. Methanol and and formaldehyde are lethal, even in very small quantities. And formaldehyde is mutagen. According to Environment Protection Agency man should not absorb more than 7.8mg of methanol per day. One liter of drink sweetened with aspartame can contain or result in 56mg of methanol[37]. That is 7 times more than suggested intake. In large quantities phenylalanine inhibits production of serotonin - a neurotransmitter.

Dangers of fluoride

Fluoride is highly toxic and was used as insecticide and rat poison. Fluoride is also a pollutant - a by-product of copper, iron and aluminum manufacturing. In 2002, nearly 90% of the U.S. population was supplied water via public water systems, and around 67% of that number received

[37] Woodrow C. Monte, Ph.D., R.D., "Aspartame: Methanol and the Public Health," Journal of Applied Nutrition

fluoridated water. Consumed in larger amounts it can actually produce tooth and bone decay, as it is non-biodegradable, and in excess can produce a condition called fluorosis, which is basically the reaction of the body to the toxin. It can come in two versions: one is calcium fluoride which is the most-common naturally-occurring form of fluoride and other is sodium fluoride which is much more dangerous.

And by study carried out from 1986 to 1987 by US National Institute of Dental Research (NIDR) on 39,207 schoolchildren, aged 5-17, in 84 areas throughout the United States found no statistically significant differences in tooth decay between people using fluoridated and non-fluoridated water[38].

The practice of water fluoridation has been rejected or banned in several countries including: China, Austria, Belgium, Finland, Germany, Denmark, Norway, Sweden, the Netherlands, Hungary, and Japan. But not in U.S.

Packaging matters

Do not consume liquids from plastic bottles at hot times as plastic releases dioxin which is highly toxic. Also do not heat your food in any sort of plastic cover in microwave as it will also release dioxin. Use ceramic or glass dishes instead.

Teflon cookware

Teflon coated cookware are easy to clean but nobody probably told you that it's toxic ! Yes you heard right, it contrains Peflourooanoic acid (PFOA) which according to EPA presents "significant developmental and reproductive risk". When Teflon® pans become sufficiently heated, the nonstick coating begins to decompose, releasing one or more of 15 different toxins. An increased rate of birth defects has been found in mothers working at DuPont. EPA even recommended that PFOA be classified as a human carcinogen. Some manufacturers mask teflon under other names such as: T-Fal, Greblon, Silverstone, Supra, and Excaliber. PFOA is also not easy to get rid of as ages can pass for detoxification.

Food additives

Like it or not, many additives are put in food to make it more "likeable". These additives are classified as "E" category in EU. It is safe to say that food containing lots of artifical additives is not healthy. Some authors claim that following additives are toxic (especially if consumed regularly) and some are even officially banned in particular countries:

E 102- Tartrazine	E-621- Monosodium Glutamate (MSG)
E 103- alkanet, alkannin	E142- Green S
E 123- Amaranth	E122- Carmoisine, Azorubine
E110-Sunset Yellow FCF	

[38] John A. Yiamouyiannis, Ph.D., „Water Fluoridation & Tooth Decay: Results from the 1986-1987 National Survey of US Schoolchildren"; http://www.fluoridealert.org/health/teeth/caries/nidr-dmft.html

(Orange Yellow S, FD&C Yellow 6)	

Important thing to have in mind here is that quantity matters. For example risk is not the same if you eat big bag of chilly potato chips from supermarket every day or once a year. So put things into perspective that risk increases exponentially the more you consume all kind of unhealthy stuff.

Free radicals&antioxidans

All basic elements (atoms) have one thing in common and that is equal number of protons in core (positively charged) and electrons in outer shell (negatively charged). Atoms that lost or gained electrons are called ions. And free radicals are nothing else than atoms with unequal number of electrons and protons which destabilize neighboring molecules. They steal electrons from neighboring atoms which in turn steal other electrons and it's a chain reaction.

One such example is oxidation, which you can best see it if you left slashed apple or banana exposed to oxygen in air. This is not to be mistaken with regulated respiration process in the cells where energy is produced.

Therefore free radical can cause mutagen processes in the DNA strand. On the other side we have antioxidants that have excess of electrons (negatively charged) and can offset influence of free radicals.

Now, there is a question of how to measure antioxidant property of particular food. Therefore ORAC (Oxygen Radical Absorbance Capacity)[39] unit, ORAC value, or "ORAC score" is a method of measuring the antioxidant capacity of different foods and supplements. It was developed by scientists at the National Institutes of Health. While the exact relationship between the ORAC value of a food and its health benefit has not directly been established, it is believed that foods higher on the ORAC scale will more effectively neutralize free radicals. According to the free-radical theory of aging, this will slow the oxidative processes and free radical damage that can contribute to age-related degeneration and disease.

So it is very important to consume food which is antioxidants to neutralize acids but also free radicals.

According to ORACValues.com food rich in antioxidants is:

Food	ORAC value
Sumac, bran, raw	312,400
Spices, cloves, ground	290,283
Sorghum, bran, hi-tannin	240,000
Spices, oregano, dried	175,295
Spices, rosemary, dried	165,280

[39] http://www.oracvalues.com/

Spices, thyme, dried	157,380
Spices, cinnamon, ground	131,420
Spices, turmeric, ground	127,068
Spices, vanilla beans, dried	122,400
Spices, sage, ground	119,929
Spices, szechuan pepper, dried	118,400
Acai, fruit pulp/skin, powder	102,700
Sorghum, bran, black	100,800
Rosehip	96,150
Sumac, grain, raw	86,800
Spices, parsley, dried	73,670
Sorghum, bran, red	71,000
Spices, nutmeg, ground	69,640
Spices, basil, dried	61,063
Cocoa, dry powder, unsweetened	55,653
Spices, cumin seed	50,372
Baking chocolate, unsweetened, squares	49,944
Spices, curry powder	48,504
Sorghum, grain, hi-tannin	45,400
Spices, pepper, white	40,700
Chocolate, dutched powder	40,200
Spices, ginger, ground	39,041
Spices, pepper, black	34,053
Sage, fresh	32,004
Spices, mustard seed, yellow	29,257
Thyme, fresh	27,426
Marjoram, fresh	27,297
Rice bran, crude	24,287
Spices, chili powder	23,636
Spices, paprika	21,932
Sorghum, grain, black	21,900
Candies, chocolate, dark	20,816
Spices, pepper, red or cayenne	19,671
Raspberries, black	19,220
Candies, semisweet chocolate	18,053
Nuts, pecans	17,940
Chokeberry, raw	16,062
Tarragon, fresh	15,542
Ginger root, raw	14,840
Elderberries, raw	14,697
Sorghum, grain, red	14,000
Peppermint, fresh	13,978
Oregano, fresh	13,970
Nuts, walnuts, english	13,541
Juice, black raspberry	10,460

Raisins, golden seedless	10,450
Nuts, hazelnuts or filberts	9,645
Blueberries, wild, raw	9,621
Pears, dried to 40% moisture (purchased in Italy)	9,496
Savory, fresh	9,465
Artichokes, Ocean Mist, boiled	9,416
Artichokes, Ocean Mist, Microwaved	9,402
Cranberries, raw	9,090
Beans, kidney, red, mature seeds, raw	8,606
Beans, black, mature seeds, raw	8,494

Source: ORACValues.com; http://www.oracvalues.com/sort/orac-value/

Other goodies

Immune-supporting vitamins and minerals can be a particularly effective approach. Vitamins A, C, B_6 and the mineral zinc are critical for optimal immune function. Vitamin A is required for the growth and activation of B-lymphocytes, increases macrophage activity, and is important in maintaining a sufficient level of natural killer cells. Deficient levels of Vitamin A can reduce lymphocyte numbers, natural killer cells, immunoglobulin responses, and impair T-lymphocyte function[40]. As mentioned earlier vitamin C is very important for immune system. It is powerfull antioxidant protecting us from oxiditve stress and is part of numerous enzymatic reactions and it is found in high concentrations in immune cells. Vitamin B_6 is important for normal immune function as deficiencies have been shown to alter lymphocyte differentiation and maturation and impair antibody production[41]. Zinc is required for normal development and function of white blood cells such as neutrophils and natural killer cells, and zinc deficiency adversely affects T-lymphocyte function, B-lymphocyte development, antibody production, and macrophage activity.

Coenzyme Q10

Coenzyme Q10 - is important because it participates in aerobic cellular respiration. And according to Dr. Warburg improper cellular respiration is prophet of cancer. Essentially it is enzyme that helps produce energy in ATP form from glucose. CoQ10 functions in every cell of the body to synthesize energy but heart, liver and kidney have the highest CoQ10 concentrations. It is widely recognized as antioxidants as well because it can easily take and give electrons. It is naturally produced by human body but additionally can be taken via pills.

Right way of eating

According to most nutritionists and some alternative practitioners animal proteins (meat, eggs, milk...) should not be consumed together with carbohydrates (wheat products, bread, rice,

---

[40] Food and Nutrition Board, Institute of Medicine. Dietary Reference Intakes for Vitamin A, Vitamin K, Arsenic, Boron, Chromium, Copper, Iodine, Iron, Manganese, Molybdenum, Nickel, Silicon, Vanadium, and Zinc. Washington, DC: National Academy Press, 2002

[41] Rall LC, Meydani SN. Vitamin B6 and immune competence. Nutr Rev. 1993 Aug

pasta…) at same time and vice versa because they require different enzymes and acidity to digest. Vegetables however are compatible with both proteins and carbohydrates.

Another important thing is to avoid consummation of solid animal fats (unmelted) as they are much harder to digest than liquid oils (sunflower, olive). Also never drink cold drinks immediately after consummation of anything containing fat as cold will solidify fat in your bowels making it also harder to digest and consequentially toxic.

Consequence of wrong diet

The following short text that describes diet related problems has been copied from Article "Cancer is a Preventable Disease that Requires Major Lifestyle Changes" published in PubMedCentral[42]:

According to an American Cancer Society study[43], obesity has been associated with increased mortality from cancers of the colon, breast (in postmenopausal women), endometrium, kidneys (renal cell), esophagus (adenocarcinoma), gastric cardia, pancreas, prostate, gallbladder, and liver. On a 900.000 sample in US the calculated risk for males to develop cancer, if obys is 52% higher and for woman risk is 62% higher.

Increased modernization and a Westernized diet and lifestyle have been associated with an increased prevalence of overweight people in many developing countries.

Heavy consumption of red meat is a risk factor for several cancers, especially for those of the gastrointestinal tract, but also for colorectal[44], prostate[45], bladder[46], breast[47], gastric[48], oral[49] cancers. Thermal preparation of meat does kill germs but can be dangerous. For example heterocyclic amines produced during the cooking of meat are carcinogens. Charcoal cooking and/or smoke curing of meat produces harmful carbon compounds such as pyrolysates and amino acids, which have a strong cancerous effect. For instance, PhIP (2-amino-1-methyl-6-phenyl-imidazo[4,5-b]pyridine) is the most abundant mutagen by mass in cooked beef and is responsible for up to 20% of

[42] Preetha Anand, Ajaikumar B. Kunnumakara, Chitra Sundaram, Kuzhuvelil B. Harikumar, Sheeja T. Tharakan, Oiki S. Lai, Bokyung Sung, and Bharat B. Aggarwal; "Cancer is a Preventable Disease that Requires Major Lifestyle Changes" published in PubMedCentral; http://www.ncbi.nlm.nih.gov/pmc/articles/PMC2515569/?tool=pmcentrez

[43] Overweight, obesity, and mortality from cancer in a prospectively studied cohort of U.S. adults; E. E. Calle, C. Rodriguez, K. Walker-Thurmond, and M. J. Thun.;

[44] S. A. Bingham, R. Hughes, and A. J. Cross. Effect of white versus red meat on endogenous N-nitrosation in the human colon and further evidence of a dose response. J. Nutr.132:3522S–3525S (2002)

A. Chao, M. J. Thun, C. J. Connell, M. L. McCullough, E. J. Jacobs, W. D. Flanders, C. Rodriguez, R. Sinha, and E. E. Calle. Meat consumption and risk of colorectal cancer. JAMA. 293:172–182 (2005) doi:10.1001/jama.293.2.172

[45] Rodriguez, M. L. McCullough, A. M. Mondul, E. J. Jacobs, A. Chao, A. V. Patel, M. J. Thun, and E. E. Calle. Meat consumption among Black and White men and risk of prostate cancer in the Cancer Prevention Study II Nutrition Cohort. Cancer Epidemiol. Biomarkers Prev. 15:211–216 (2006)

[46] R. Garcia-Closas, M. Garcia-Closas, M. Kogevinas, N. Malats, D. Silverman, C. Serra, A. Tardon, A. Carrato, G. Castano-Vinyals, M. Dosemeci, L. Moore, N. Rothman, and R. Sinha. Food, nutrient and heterocyclic amine intake and the risk of bladder cancer. Eur. J. Cancer. 43:1731–1740 (2007)

[47] A. Tappel. Heme of consumed red meat can act as a catalyst of oxidative damage and could initiate colon, breast and prostate cancers, heart disease and other diseases. Med. Hypotheses. 68:562–4 (2007)

[48] L. H. O'Hanlon. High meat consumption linked to gastric-cancer risk. Lancet Oncol. 7:287 (2006)

[49] T. N. Toporcov, J. L. Antunes, and M. R. Tavares. Fat food habitual intake and risk of oral cancer.

the total mutagenicity found in fried beef. Daily intake of PhIP among Americans is estimated to be 280–460 ng/day per person[50].

Nitrites and nitrates are used in meat because they bind to myoglobin, inhibiting botulinum exotoxin production; however, they are powerful carcinogens[51]. Long-term exposure to food additives such as nitrite preservatives and azo dyes has been associated with the induction of carcinogenesis[52]. Furthermore, bisphenol from plastic food containers can migrate into food and may increase the risk of breast[53] and prostate[54] cancers. Ingestion of arsenic may increase the risk of bladder, kidney, liver, and lung cancers[55]. Saturated fatty acids, trans fatty acids, and refined sugars and flour present in most foods have also been associated with various cancers. Several food carcinogens have been shown to activate inflammatory pathways.

Bad diet, physical inactivity, and obesity altogether are related to approximately 30–35% of cancer cases. In the United States excess body weight is associated with the development of many types of cancer and is a factor in 14–20% of all cancer deaths[56].

Detoxification

At the end of food chain we come to question of detoxification. We absorb nutrients from food but toxic compounds builds up in our bodies and are being increasingly recognized as common cause of cancer.

This can happen for two obvious reasons:

a) excess toxic intake via food and water

b) inability of body to flush out toxins

Some authors, like Norman Walker, recognized importance of detoxification many decades ago. He has written great deal of books on the matter and you are certainly advised to read them. Bottom of this logic is that toxics, usually because of excess meat or carbohydrates, build up in your colon and with years your body is unable to expel them and they simply rot there spreading

---

[50] S. N. Lauber, and N. J. Gooderham. The cooked meat derived genotoxic carcinogen 2-amino-3-methylimidazo[4,5-b]pyridine has potent hormone-like activity: mechanistic support for a role in breast cancer.

[51] D. Divisi, S. Di Tommaso, S. Salvemini, M. Garramone, and R. Crisci. Diet and cancer. Acta Biomed. 77:118–123 (2006)

[52] Y. F. Sasaki, S. Kawaguchi, A. Kamaya, M. Ohshita, K. Kabasawa, K. Iwama, K. Taniguchi, and S. Tsuda. The comet assay with 8 mouse organs: results with 39 currently used food additives. Mutat. Res.519:103–119 (2002)

[53] M. Durando, L. Kass, J. Piva, C. Sonnenschein, A. M. Soto, E. H. Luque, and M. Munoz-de-Toro. Prenatal bisphenol A exposure induces preneoplastic lesions in the mammary gland in Wistar rats. Environ. Health Perspect.115:80–6 (2007).

[54] S. M. Ho, W. Y. Tang, J. Belmonte de Frausto, and G. S. Prins. Developmental exposure to estradiol and bisphenol A increases susceptibility to prostate carcinogenesis and epigenetically regulates phosphodiesterase type 4 variant 4. Cancer Res.66:5624–32 (2006)

[55] A. Szymanska-Chabowska, J. Antonowicz-Juchniewicz, and R. Andrzejak. Some aspects of arsenic toxicity and carcinogenicity in living organism with special regard to its influence on cardiovascular system, blood and bone marrow. Int. J. Occup. Med. Environ. Health. 15:101–116 (2002).

[56] A. Drewnowski, and B. M. Popkin. The nutrition transition: new trends in the global diet. Nutr. Rev.55:31–43 (1997).

---

toxicity all round. Therefore it is quite essential to perform colon cleansing every so often and combine this with strict diet consisting only of freshly squeezed juices that will replenish your nutrient reserves. Colon cleansing may be considered impractical and repulsive thing to do in clinic but you can also perform it in your house using intake of 50g of magnesium salt for two days.

Mr. Walker claims he cured dozens of people suffering from all kind of diseases this way and that state of affairs of particular part of your colon can have direct consequences on corresponding organs in entire body as suggested by following picture:

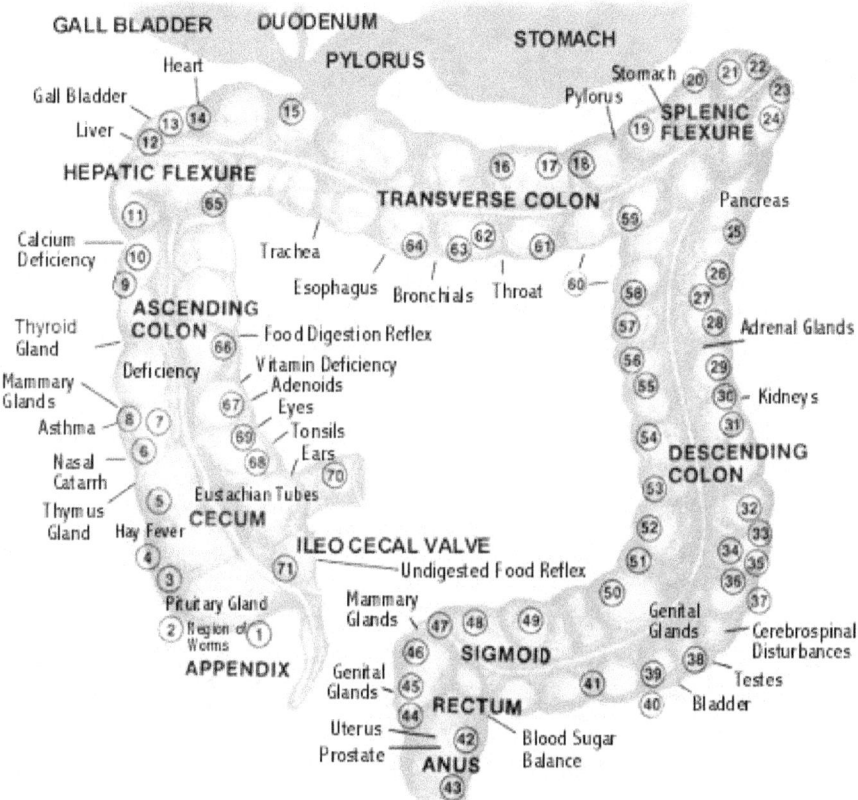

What does this mean and what should I do ?

There are several things here more than worth mentioning. First is to moderately consume animal proteins. Preferably from animals that are not stuffed with all kind of hormones and antibiotics and which were fed properly. Second is to cut down carbohydrates as much as possible as they will clog your body from start to finish. Third is to avoid sugary products as cancer cells have are extremely dependent on glucose and ferment sugar. Impact of sugar on immune system also seems to be horrifying. Overall, this text provides more than enough bridges between sugar and cancer.

Fourth is that you obviously need to eat more vegetables, nuts and berries which are usually alkaline and have antioxidants properties as to partly replace previous three kinds. Fifth is that you need to drink as much of fresh juice from vegetables and fruit. And by fresh I mean no more than 15 min old. By eating right food you not only provide fuel of adequate quality to your cells, but you also hopefully cut-out numerous toxins previously digested. Furthermore you alkalize your body increasing it's oxygen burning capabilities.

Sixth is that you need to regularly clean your body via feasting on fresh juices and performing colon cleansing from time to time.

4. Stress

Human body is extremely complicated electro - chemical machine. It consists of several critical systems necessary to sustain life like:

- cardiovascular system
- nervous system
- digestion system
- muscular and bone system
- etc.

Each of this is composed of organs and highly specialized tissues which are usually very sensitive to outside shocks. We mentioned earlier that every material when put under sufficient stress - breaks. The question is just how much stress. Stress disturbs this fine electro - chemical balance in human body.

Stressors can be anything from your perception of reality, ranging from annoying member of your family to buzzing sound disturbing your sleep. So one can suffer stress at home, work and host of other locations. Stress can leave behind visible and invisible consequences. Usually consequences are invisible until lot's of them pilled up to result in physical or mental disease. Therefore timely detection of stressors can't be voiced more important.

People who suffer from stress usually are not concentrated, have memory problems, don't sleep well, have bad perspective of life, are nervous and agitated etc. But in sufficient quantity stress can also cause or accelerate development of malignant processes. Think about it like this, stress or it's manifestation like fear, anger and other powerful emotions can cause surge in hormones, enzymes, adrenalin in your blood or neurotransmitters like dopamine. This is NOT normal and should be avoided at all costs. Adrenaline alone should be used only for life threatening situations and not misused for day to day stressors. Although this, by itself may not directly and instantly cause cancer it certainly decreases our immune system, making us more vulnerable to all kind of disruptions not excluding cancerous developments.

Also, stress causes no enviable amount of mental diseases or disorders that require psychiatric help. All this is also happening on cellular level and is by no means healthy.

The important thing, like with everything in life is to learn how to manage it. And management means three things:

1. Identify stressor

2. Learn how to ignore or lower influence of stressor or, ultimately, accept stressors point of view so you avoid further conflict

3. If actions under point 2 can't be done cut all links with stressor whatsoever

Usually the people have problems at work with colleagues or with inadequate salary or with wedding partner whom they grew tired of. If salary is the problem and you can't cover all expenses, rather than despair try cutting down all costs except basic life supporting things. And coffee with donut 5 times a day is by no means life supporting. Remember, if it's not life supporting you don't need it. No money is worth eroding your health as no money will repair it afterwards. If work is the problem try changing working environment, dial up some old friends for connections and check with local bureau if there is another working place available for your qualifications. If it's your marriage than it's a bit of more of a problem especially with children involved. But if daily fights can't be avoided it's better to call it quits and start over - because if things don't improve you are only guaranteed with a failure. And wasting time on failure is no way to go forward. You may be better of trying to find a success than constantly trying to reinforce a failure. Human beings were not meant to be psychologically tormented on daily basis.

Therefore stress is heavily connected with psychology ie. state of mind. If you can't sleep, if you are not at peace with yourself or with others you are suffering some sort of stress and have a bad thing coming. Sooner or later consequences will show. Life without debt and without other life threatening dangers should enable peace of mind which harmonizes delicate electro-chemical processes necessary to sustain our body and life. Positive outlook on life, which is certainly justified in majority of situations, is extremely important for human health. Just how psychic influences our immune system is yet to be fully explained by scientists but we know that cortisol, released from the adrenal glands, is the primary hormone that mediates the stress response and suppresses the immune response.[10]

Research has shown that stress can affect the immune system in several ways such as reduced neutrophil activity, changes in types of chemical mediators (cytokines) produced by the white blood cells, and decreased cytotoxic T-lymphocytes and natural killer cell activities[57]. Studies suggest that an elevated cortisol:DHEA ratio is a contributing factor to this reduced immunity, particularly in elderly patients. DHEA (dehydroepiandrosterone) is a steroid hormone secreted from the adrenal glands). More specifically, an elevated cortisol:DHEA ratio significantly decreases neutrophil activity.

Importance of sleep

Deep sleep naturally heals our body and alleviates stress. It is especially good for resting the mind. After 8 hours of good sleep everyone will feel refreshed. The problem only is how fast will "junk" be poured into that mind again. Sleep deprivation is serious problem as it does not provide chance to our body to do what it is intended to do. Sleep deprivation decreases strength of immune system. If somebody suffers from insomnia, hard physical labor and fresh air can help. When physically exhausted our body immediately yearns for good sleep to decrease level of lactic acid created by physical activity.

---

[57] Reiche EM, Morimoto HK, Nunes SM. Stress and depression-induced immune dysfunction: implications for the development and progression of cancer. Int Rev Psychiatry. 2005 Dec;

What does this mean and what should I do ?

Stress ultimately causes illnesses either mental or physical. Or both. But you may not recognize it for some time, maybe until it's too late. Propensity to stress depends hugely on type of personality you are. Some people are itchy by nature and are annoyed even by minor things. Yet another kind of people fails or ignores to take notice of even obvious occasions such as birthdays or bills that should be paid each month. Don't be annoyed by minor and insignificant things and let things flow their own way - you don't have to influence everything. If a college gets promoted instead of you, don't take it too seriously and go on as usual. If a loyal friend sleeps with your partner, think soberly for couple of days and make a clear cut decision with sober head without recriminations afterwards. Don't eat yourself up over things you can't change. If you are subject to harassment or psychological torture at home or at work, clearly define situation as such and take necessary steps. This should be of such nature that in future reflections you don't look back at yourself with a pity.

Also accept that some things are as they are, even if maybe a bit unfair. Not all creatures are created equal nor are all things balanced, nor rights equal justice, nor are all matters right, nor is it up to you to always make them right. Nor do we always have information even to judge what is right and what is wrong.

Number of stress reducing therapies exists. One is yoga for example, which help individuals do a bit of soul searching and help find necessary inner peace. This inner peace is connected with happiness and positive outlook on life. Others methods include simple things like listening to relaxing music (waves of oceans, forest sounds, Tibetan drums etc.) which can easily be found on video portals like YouTube and are free.

5. Genetics

Cancers are caused by changes to materials in our bodies called "genes." These genes are part of DNA strand. Some genes tell our bodies how to fix damage accumulated over time from normal aging, environmental toxins, sun exposure, dietary factors, hormones, and other influences. When genes themselves are damaged, they can develop changes called "mutations." When mutations occur in the damage-controlling genes, cells can grow out of control and cause cancer. For most people who develop cancer, the cancer-causing gene mutations happen over the course of a lifetime, leading to cancer later in life. Some people are born with a gene mutation that they inherited from their mother or father. This damaged gene puts them at higher risk for cancer than most people. People with an inherited gene change have a 50% chance of passing the mutation to each of their children.[58]

The vast majority of cancers are non-hereditary ("sporadic cancers"). Hereditary cancers are primarily caused by an inherited genetic defect. Less than 0.3% of the population is carrier of a genetic mutation which has a large effect on cancer risk and this cause less than 3–10% of all cancers[59]. Some of these syndromes include: certain inherited mutations in the genes BRCA1 and BRCA2 with a more than 75% risk of breast cancer and ovarian cancer, and hereditary nonpolyposis colorectal cancer (HNPCC or Lynch syndrome) which is present in about 3% of people with colorectal cancer, among others[60].

What does this mean and what should I do ?

Genetic counseling is available. Genetic counselors discuss your family history in depth and determine your risk factor. Depending on your cancer family history, the counselor can recommend genetic testing. It is recommended that if you have several family members who have had the same cancer, such as breast cancer, to seek genetic counseling. There is a simple blood test that can detect a mutated BRCA gene. People can also take PSA test for prostate cancer or detailed genetic test laboratory tests of DNA for mutated MLH1 and MSH2 genes in colorectal cancer.

---

[58] http://www.facingourrisk.org/info_research/hereditary-cancer/hereditary-genetics/index.php

[59] Roukos, DH (2009). "Genome-wide association studies: how predictable is a person's cancer risk?"

[60] Cunningham, D; Atkin, W, Lenz, HJ, Lynch, HT, Minsky, B, Nordlinger, B, Starling, N (2010 Mar 20) "Colorectal cancer."

II. "Official" and "alternative" explanations and treatments of cancer

A lot has been said so far of possible cancer causes. And they are all valid as logic is concerned. However, oncologists (alternatives call them pathologists) around the world are not unanimous what exactly can cause cancer, neither they want to bother much with causes. They simply define cancer as "uncontrolled tissue growth" and have several standard methods of dealing with it once it occurs as is the case with every other disease.

Alternatives on the other hand are even more dispersed and disorganized as there are literally dozens of ideas what causes cancer and how it should be cured. Some prominent figures believe it is caused by tiny parasites (yeast included) and have some unique ways of dealing with them. This book will not go into extreme details and exact dosages of each and every alternative treatment (although overview of major treatments will be provided) and author of this book neither promotes nor opposes use of alternative treatments. However, one objective of this book was to describe some natural and cheap ways to prevent and treat cancer.

And what is patient to do ?

It is important to understand here that you, dear reader, are ruler of your destiny. And nobody can take you that right, neither medical institution, neither your doctor. First, a patient has **a right to information**. To me it's striking that people on chemotherapy are not presented with statistics about success rate of such terrible treatment in particular case of cancer. Doctors are not gods. They have to do what is prescribed by medical protocols in order to protect themselves and won't go into much discussion how effective particular treatment will be in each case. In many cases aforementioned chemotherapy severely destroys immune system which each person should be well aware of it in advance as it is questionable whether this warning will be put forward by respective oncologist. But one needs that information in order to decide whether will he stick with for chemotherapy which is almost useless for lets say melanoma (IV stage) or will he decide to undergo alternative treatments which are usually painless but also with variable results.

Question of time

For cancer patients, time is running out. Usually quite fast. So decisions which are made must be made in good time. I will give just one example. If cancer is detected early it's good to have it remove via surgery and not risk with alternative protocols. If it metastasizes the problem is 1000 times bigger and 1000 times more expansive. If cancer has spread around official medicine will prescribe massive surgery, chemotherapy or immunotherapy which may or may not work. It is in these cases patients often look out for alternative medicine.

Question of money

Late detected cancer cases and HIV patients usually shell out between 10.000$ and 500.000$ for their treatments. If we multiply that with number of new cancer cases we come to some staggering numbers and start to grasp the size of this business. This is big industry with even bigger profits and shareholders. Companies earn loads on chemotherapy, immunotherapy (interleukin, interferon), or HIV suppression drugs. So unless you have pretty good insurance policy you are facing some heavy investments down the road. Cases are not rare when patients sold houses to pay for treatment. Alternative medicine on the other hand is usually dirt cheap. But as always decision is on patient which way he chooses.

Question of principle

"Official" medicine sticks with principle of slash (surgery), burn (radiation) or poison (chemotherapy). It does not look at causes of cancer whatsoever. Chemotherapy for example works by destroying all fast growing cells, including red and white blood cells.

"Alternative" medicine usually looks at causes of cancer and relies heavily on persons own immune system and tries to strengthen it via various natural supplements. It also tries to find substances which inhibit or destroy cancer cells (like Aloe Vera or Laetrille). "Alternative" medicine even includes some exotic measures like induced hyperthermia (rising of body temperature) as this was proven to adversely affect cancer cells by a study of Royal College of Surgeons of England in 1974 ![61] This treatment is actually officially applied in Germany but not in USA so its questionable where to drawn the line between alternative and "official" medicine.

---

[61] Annals of the Royal College of Surgeons of England (1974) vol 54

1. "Official" explanation and treatment of cancer

Cancer is officially described as uncontrolled tissue growth. It requires modification of genes that regulate cell division like growth suppressor genes (which cancel cell division when something has gone wrong). However for tumor to develop changes is several genes are usually required. In mitosis improper replication of chromosome can occur while damage from various sources can damage DNA strand itself at any time.

Cancers are usually classified by the type of cell they grow in and are divided as follows:

Reproduction cancer: testicle or the ovary cancer.

Sarcoma: Cancers of connective tissue i.e. bone, and nerve cancer.

Carcinoma: Affect epithelial cells. Includes breast, prostate, lung, pancreas, and colon cancer.

Lymphoma and leukemia: They appear in lymph nodes and blood.

Official medicine also recognizes following cases of cancer treatment:

Surgery

Most common method of cancer treatment. Biopsies are usually required. Surgeon removes entire tissue affected area. Usually it is used in combination with other methods like chemotherapy and radiation. It is almost applicable to wide range of cancers cases. Some cancers may seem localized but spread around in lymph, so lymph nods are also often removed. And there is great deal of them in human body.

Does it makes sense ?

Yes, especially if cancer is detected in early stage and is localized. However if it has spread around surrounding tissue via metastasis, chemotherapy may be the only thing left as official medicine is concerned.

Chemotherapy

Chemotherapy is applied when surgery is not enough or it does not provide assurance cancer that enough cells have been removed. It is applicable to cancer of most internal organs like ovarian cancer, breast cancer, colorectal cancer, pancreatic cancer, sarcoma, testicular cancer and lung cancers. Negative side is that chemotherapy is toxic to human tissue and can't be applied indefinitely.

Side-effects affect all cells that are fast growing like patient's hair follicles, their bone marrow, and the cells lining the stomach and intestines.

Does it makes sense ?

It does to certain degree and for certain types of cancer, especially if cancer has spread around via metastasis. Surgeons can only cut tissue to a point and it would make no sense in radiating entire body to catch all metastasis. Therefore chemotherapy seems like only logical solution. But results vary horribly, and that is why you must get pretty informed before undergoing this kind of treatment.

Radiation

Radiation therapy applies ionizing radiation to kill as much cancer cells as possible. As is the case with chemotherapy it also has downsides that include radiation of all cells that fall under radiation beam meaning healthy cells are killed or modified also.

Does it makes sense ?

Yes, if cancer is localized and surgery is not applicable. This is certainly more preferable to chemotherapy.

Immunotherapy

Oncologists will sometimes decide for patient to undergo other type of therapy and that is immunotherapy which is aimed at strengthening immune system. It is usually done by administering interleukin and interferon both of which are usual part of everyone's immune system. These kinds of therapies are extremely expensive and are applied in rare cases.

2. "Alternative" explanation and treatment of cancer

Since the time began all kind of people tried to cure all kind of diseases. Sometimes they were successful and their practices were adopted in "official" medicine. Alternative practitioners usually try to cure cancer using natural substances and methods and are therefore called naturopaths. These kinds of practices are legal or illegal or are in "grey zone" depending on the country at hand. But there is bigger, even ideological struggle to consider. Usually alternative practitioners consider medical associations as cartels whose sole purpose is to sell as much expansive cures which do not work. Robert Beck coined this nicely: "patient cured is customer lost".

Again it must be stressed out that decision to rest your life with alternative treatments is your decision and must be based on adequate information which at least should include:

a) what are your chances with "official" treatments like chemotherapy

b) what are chances that particular alternative treatment will work

There are some restrictions here, as some patients are in such condition as not able to digest food. These should pay special attention to methods of alternative treatment.

Alternative practitioners are by no means unanimous or coherent group or better to say most prominent figures have their "own way" of dealing with cancer. Some foremost alternative practitioners are or better to say were: Dr. Royal Riffe, Dr. Bob Beck, Norman Walker, Dr. Hulda Clark, Dr. Tulio Simoccini etc. They usually developed their own protocols for healing cancer.

Alternatives got going in 1930s when Dr. Warburg discovered that oxygen starvation is critical to cancer development. His work was superseded by Dr. Budwig who found out that cancer patients have unusually low levels of unsaturated fatty acids in blood which in turn prevents proper oxygen supply and transport to cells. She also had great success and became famous for so called "Budwig diet" including cottage cheese and flax seed to make up for deficiency of unsaturated fatty acids in blood.

Along these lines came Norman Walker who became world famous for his theories on proper diet consisting of fresh juices and salads. His advices may be ridiculed but nobody on official medicaments came close to live 113 years as Norman did !

Dr. Tulio Simoccini became famous by claiming that Candida Albicans (form of yeast) causes cancer and for devising very simple cure – sodium bicarbonate. He apparently cured many patients with intravenous injection of sodium carbonate solution.

Dr. William Donald Kelley claimed that cancers are result of enzyme deficiency. He apparently cured thousands of cancer patents many of whom official medicine has given up. He put them on special diet and made sure they are given sufficient enzymes. Enzymes excreted pancreas and liver dissolve cancer protein as well as protein from food. A rule popped up here that meat and proteins should not be consumed throughout the day as enzymes are used up in digestion. Therefore proteins should be eaten only for lunch and thereby use up enzymes for 4 hours instead of 12 or 16 hours a day. He also has unique explanation that cancer is nothing more than primitive germ cell (pre-placenta cells) growing normally in the wrong place and there are about 2 of these germ cells in for every 10 cubic mm of our body.

Dr. Lorrain Day cured herself of cancer and written nice material of how proper diet looks like.

Overall, we can classify these alternative practitioners into three groups:

a) ones that think oxygen deprivation is cause of cancer

b) ones that believe that enzyme and nutrients deficiency cause cancer

c) ones that believe that parasite infection causes cancer and are to be treated with electromagnetic fields and electrical current

The third group is especially interesting because no small number of patents exists on this and similar subjects and all came to light because of Dr. Robert Beck in 1993. But before going into this we must mention work of Dr. Royal Raymond Rife who was self-thought in many natural sciences and devised some ingenious solution for cancer problem. He was microbiologist and among first to claim that cancer is caused by parasites and that all parasites, bacteria, viruses and pathogens can be destroyed by radio waves tuned to particular frequency. Apparently he had great success and cured all 16 cancer patients in clinical trial that took place in California in 1934, but his practices were later banned by Federal and Drug Administration.

Following his steps Dr. Robert Beck discovered that leading American universities have in 1993 patented cure for AIDS through electrical treatment of blood. In patent No. 5,188,738 it was mentioned that this process "attenuates all know viruses, including HIV" and "does not make blood unfit for use in humans". Dr. Beck than devised very cheap instrument called "zapper" that induces 50miliAmpers of electrical current in blood via electrodes strapped to hand wrist arteries and changing frequency at 4Hz which destroys HIV and other viruses. Patent No. 4,665,898 describes how magnetic field can be successfully used to treat cancer. AND THAT MUST BE A SURPRISE - THAT CHEAP CURE FOR HIV AND CANCER IS PATENTED.

Patent No. 5091152 describes exactly how bacteria E. Colli can be totally destroyed by electrical current of 350miliAmpers at frequency of 1800 Hz and waveform of particular shape.

Following this he realized that magnetic fields can destroy cancer cells and consequentially designed so called Magnetic pulsar which is able to penetrate deep tissue (few inches) like lymph and internal organs and destroy parasites there. He also reinvented "colloidal silver" which in combination with zapper destroys all fungus, bacteria and viruses in blood. So he effectively combined patents for cure on HIV and cancer in something that is called Bob Beck protocol which is described later.

Now, if we take into account fact that Papiloma virus surely can cause uterus cancer than this viewpoint should not be taken lightly or to say it otherwise, parasite and virus infection can possibly lead to cancer and if that is the case it can almost certainly be destroyed by electromagnetic fields of particular frequency (publicized by Dr. Royal Rife) and electrical current (publicized by Dr. Robert Beck).

This is similar to what Royal Riffe was claiming and proved almost a century ago before he was banned. From this origins conspiracy theory emerged saying patients today are slaves of medical establishment who is in fact not interested to cure patients but to rip them off as much as possible.

One other thing must be said here and that is that Riffe, Beck and others thought cancer cells can be reverted back to normal cells whereas "official" medicine excludes this possibility outright. They more/less proved that once parasites are destroyed, cells indeed continue to function normally, they don't ferment glucose anymore and don't replicate constantly. They argue that their electrocution certainly does not repair damaged DNA but almost certainly kills parasites.

Dr. Hulda Clark followed up on his steps, devising a zapper of her own but working on slightly different principles.

When talking about electricity we must mention Dr. Parker who was German and Austrian physician. He developed methods of erasing malignant growths based on the use of electricity ie. applying low voltage current via electrodes directly to tumor area. And this had great success. This practice was consequentially conveyed to China who, unlike USA, was very interested. Results did not fall short. At the Second International Conference of Bio-Electrotherapy for Cancer held in Stockholm, Sweden, in 1993, the Chinese oncological participants reported that their administration of BET to 4,000 cancer patients resulted in an accumulation of Complete Remissions and Partial Remissions (CR+PR) exceeding 80%.

As with other natural treatments, Dr. Parker says there is no money to be made in this effective treatment. As usual there is patent on this issue No. 7204834 patented in 2007 which claims electric currents (heal cancer.

It is interesting that all of alternative practitioners had considerable success in treating cancer cases many of which were already given up by official medicine. As usual internet is biggest library on these issues and dear reader is certainly advised to goggle up any topic of particular importance and most important have been presented here.

As alternative websites are concerned special mention must go to Independent Cancer Research Foundation, Inc. (ICRF) at Cancertutor.com[62] (and its founder Webster Kehr) which is probably best collection of alternative cancer medicine on web. There you can find various protocols, dosages, substances and treatments.

Other great source of info can be found at Dr. Kelley web page:
http://www.drkelley.com/CANLIVER55.html

---

[62] www.cancertutor.com

3. Mostly used protocols/treatments

Bob Beck protocol

This protocol implicitly presumes that cancer is caused by parasites and they should be treated as such. It consists of four devices:

- electrical zapper – which is intended to destroy parasites in blood by inducing electrical current via electrodes strapped on a hand wrist arteries. It should be worn for 2 hors daily.

- magnetic pulsar – which is intended to destroy parasites hiding in deeper organs and lymph nodes via powerful magnetic fields. It should be applied for 2 hors daily.

- colloidal silver – which is proven to destroy bacteria, viruses in blood etc. It should be drunk after pulsing and zapping to destroy remnants in blood and purify it.

- ozone water – which also oxidizes cancer tissue and kills parasites. It should be drunk before and after pulsing and zapping to destroy remnants in blood and purify it.

There are wonderful materials on this subject and reader is certainly advised to look them in more detail. Word of warning is appropriate here as patients should stop intake of all supplements and drug 2 days before starting with electrical zapper because it increases propensity of your blood to carry substances.

Flax seed oil protocol

The Flaxseed (Linseed) oil diet was originally proposed by Dr. Johanna Budwig, a German biochemist and expert on fats and oils, in 1951 and recently re-examined by Dr. Dan C. Roehm M.D. FACP (Oncologist and former cardiologist) in 1990. Dr. Roehm claims: "this diet is far and away the most successful anti-cancer diet in the world".

Budwig claims that the diet is both a preventative and a curative. She says the absence of linol-acids [in the average western diet] is responsible for the production of oxydase, which induces cancer growth and is the cause of many other chronic disorders. Dr. Johanna Budwig cured hundreds of cancer patients this way and claims success rate was 90% in few months.

The beneficial oxydase ferments are destroyed by heating or boiling oils in foods, and by nitrates used for preserving meat, etc. The theory is: the use of oxygen in the organism can be stimulated by protein compounds of sulphuric content, which make oils water-soluble and which is present in cheese, nuts, onion and leek vegetables such as leek, chive, onion and garlic, but especially cottage cheese. Ferments of cell respiration closely connected with the highly unsaturated fatty acids that are also needed for proper oxidation. Unprocessed flax seed oil provides two essential fatty acid which are deficient in Western diet: 1) Linolenic acid and 2) Linoleic acid. These two unsaturated fatty acids have three high energy double bonds in their electron shells. This fatty acids enable big increase in oxygen assimilation. By substantially increasing oxidation potential

Dr. Budwig confirmed what Dr. Warburg had discovered before that cancer can't survive in oxygen rich environment.

A person requires daily about 4 oz. of cottage cheese mixed well with 1.5 oz. of linseed oil and 1 oz. of milk. A blender or egg beater works fine. The mixture can be sweeten with honey or otherwise flavored naturally. Fresh fruits can be added. Every morning 2 spoonfuls of freshly ground linseed oil should be taken in warm buttermilk or yoghurt.

Protocol envisages mixing of cottage cheese with flax seed in 3:1 ration. You can put in fresh juice or champagne. Instead of cottage cheese you can use yogurt. Should be mixed in blender for few mins so no oil is visible and as suh is much easier to digest.

Protocol also describes that you should not eat any meat and ban all sugar while on protocol. And drink lots of fresh juices and liquid. Also consuming freshly crushed Flax oil seed (6 spoon a day) is very important as it contains nutrients not present in Flax seed oil. You can mix them in blender.

Amygdalin (Laetrile):

When the natural substance called amygdalin is purified and concentrated for use in cancer therapy, it is called Laetrile. Amygdalin is extracted from apricot seeds and prepared in both tablet and injectable form. It is usually recommended at the onset of treatment for patients who are seriously ill. It can be taken if form of tablets, solution or apricot seeds. This therapy is usually used in conjunction with the proteolytic enzymes, a broad-spectrum nutritional program, and a diet calling for fresh fruits and vegetables, whole grains, and the elimination of meat and dairy products for the duration of treatment. Official medicine discards amygdalin as cancer treatment substance quoting it has not been proven in clinical testing.

Usual therapy includes 10 apricot seeds+table spoon of latrille solution (or tablet equivalent) 3 times a day. With laetrile its crucial to take zinc and proteolytic enzymes. Theraphy lasts for 2 weeks than 1 week off and than again 2 weeks on.

There are case of isolated ethnic tribes like Navajo Indians, the Hunzas the Abkhasians and who had consume large quantities of Apricot Kernels (Amygdalin) and had no reported cases of cancer. One of the most common nitrilosides is amygdalin.

Aloe vera

Father Fr. Romano Zago's discovered it's healing properties in Brazil. It helps the body fight infections and malignant cells. It is also a detoxifier and an immunomodulator, meaning it will raise your immune system. It requires special production process. It is to be harvested only after 5 years, crushed and mixed with low concentration alcohol and kept out of sunlight. So be aware of various Aloe Vera related marketing products, because they are usually just marketing. Theraphy usually lasts for 3 weeks than 1 week off. 1 spoon is consumed 3 times a day, and no meat should be digested meanwhile.

Enzyme supplement protocol

Dr. Kelley is proponent of the idea that cancer shows up when our capacity to produce enzymes falls down ie. when we age. He says that enzymes designed to dissolve animal protein (as used in digestion) also can dissolve cancer tissue which is protein as well. Therefore no meat should be consumed except for lunch and various cocktail of enzymes needs to be administered usually in form of pills. Trypsin enzyme break down tumor mass and is opposite to cancer producing enzyme malignin which breaks down human protein. Enzyme Serrapeptase, found in supplements such as Vitalzyme, is shown to actively tears down thick cancer cells membrane which prevent white blood cells and immune system to destroy cancer.

Sodium bicarbonate (iodine)

Dr. Tulio Simoccini is founder of idea that cancer is caused by yeast "Albina Candida". Good thing is that this yeast can be easily destroyed with cheap substance called sodium bicarbonate which also strongly alkalizes our body. Exact dosages vary depending on type of cancer and they should be looked upon his site http://www.curenaturalicancro.com

Iodine - iodine is known in medicine as disinfectant and antiseptic. Table salt is usually iodized for needs of our thyroid gland. Italian Dr. Simocini suggests that iodine is used for exclusive treatment of skin cancers.

There are numerous live testimonials on his website http://www.curenaturalicancro.com/cancer-therapy-video.html about patients who were given up on by official medicine but were cured with his iodine treatments. He recommends 7% iodine solution to be applied 20 times a day for five days with 10 day break.

Electrocution

German and an Austrian physician, Dr. Pekar developed methods of erasing malignant growths based on the use of electricity ie. applying low voltage current via electrodes directly to tumor area. The dosage is a few milliamperes which are applied for up to 90 minutes via ordinary 9 volt battery. In order to understand the mechanism of cancer cells and the fact that they are "masked" from the immune system, one has to look deeper into the functioning of bioelectric currents. An electric voltage is part of all functions in living tissue. It arises primarily at the cellular walls and gives rise to electric currents. Cell membranes contain ion channels. They carry a negative charge at the outside of the cell membrane and show selectivity for kations, particularly for sodium and potassium ions. Part of these ion channels open only after adequate change of the membrane potential. Cell life depends on the nutritional input and adequate excretion of metabolic end products. Both pathways use the ion channels. This metabolism constitutes the flow of electric current. If a cell does not function normally, it emits an electromagnetic field which differs from the healthy field condition. Cancer cells carry a negative membrane potential which is proportional to the degree of their malignancy. This change in potential enables the cell to separate from other cells and to maintain its masking capabilities towards the reconnaissance function of the immune system. The cell's altered protein metabolism produces a membrane attacking enzyme which enables it to penetrate and to infiltrate normal surrounding tissue. Cell resonance changes and the dynamic condition of tissue is being destroyed through polarity change[63]. After applying current, energetic ionic flow of current is re-established at the same time in accordance with the naturally intended structure of the organism.

Sending electric currents through tumor tissue leads to electrolytic changes at the electrodes which in turn causes significant alterations of the pH value. As that pH value differs from the normal physiological range it will be destructive for tumor tissue. The results show an aseptic necrosis of tissue and an accompanying "unmasking" of the cancer cells now made recognizable to the immune system. Cancer cells caught between the positive and negative poles depolarize, so they become permeable and accept various substances that are poisonous to them.

The phagocytic cells (stimulated where required via additional immunotherapy) will break down and destroy the dead remnants of the tumor within one to three weeks.

The process is best applied in respective clinic (mandatory in case of non-skin tumors) or by physician and usually lasts for 30-90 minutes each day for several weeks or until tumor is in remission.

Grape Cure

We all know grape cure is powerful antioxidant, but few know it can be used to treat cancer. It was invented in 1920s by Johanna Brandt. Protocol is divided in two 12-12 hours period. Patient eats nothing but grapes (with skin and seeds) for 12 hours from, say, 9 am to 9 pm and fasts at all other times. Naturally it consumes ONLY pure water (not distilled nor chlorinated) as water incites cancer cells to eat up glucose in grape. However, aside glucose, grape has many other cancer killing substances which get consumed as well.

Cesium chloride

Cesium is one of most alkaline elements and logic of it's application follows logic of previously described pH. As was stated, it is believed, that cancer cells can't survive in high pH environment. Cancer cells absorb elements various elements. Potassium ions are responsible for the ability of glucose to enter the cell. Calcium, magnesium and sodium ions, which are responsible for the intake of oxygen into the cell, can not enter the cancer cell but the potassium ion still enters these cells[64]. The most alkaline minerals (cesium, rubidium, potassium) are able to enter cancer cells.

Dr H. E. Sartori had great success with cesium treatments in April 1981 at Life Sciences Universal Medical Clinics in Rockville. He treated 50 terminal patients with various cancers and almost 50% of patients survived. Physicist A. Keith Brewer in 1930s treated 30 patients with cesium and all survived.

Some take it together with substance called DMSO (Dimethyl sulfoxide). This is especially the case if normal digestion of patient is impaired. DMSO can than greatly help in trans-dermal transfer of cesium through skin. Word of warning, however, consumption of cesium depletes body reserves of magnesium and potassium which therefore must be taken as additional supplements. Excess cesium can have severe consequences on human body and death was reported in several cases because of heart arrhythmia. When consuming cesium, levels of potassium and magnesium in body must be monitored every 2 weeks.

[63] http://www.healingcancernaturally.com/greatesthits4.html

[64] http://www.newswithviews.com/Howenstine/james14.htm

Exact dosages are prescribed by Wolf-clinic[65] and say 1.5 g of cesium is consumed three times a in a spoon after meal. It is taken for five days than two days, than again five days, two days off for a period of 4 weeks. Cesium stays in human body for 3 months before being flushed out, so once "cesium limit" is hit, another round of cesium protocol can't be administered for period of at least 3 months. Transdermal protocol consists of mixing cesium with DMSO and water in ratio 1:1:1. Some people may be allergic to DMSO and therefore smaller doses should be applied first.

Some might argue why deals with this unnatural substances, but they forget that if somebody is dying of cancer that person should have right of choice how to help himself.

Hyperthermia

Hyperthermia is not such a novel idea as supposedly president Regan underwent this treatment in Germany in 1980-is. And this treatment is usual practice in Germany today. But it can't be applied legally in USA. It's concept is founded on the fact that elevated temperature levels ranging from 106-113F (39-42 Celsius) destroys cancer cells as proven by the a study of Royal College of Surgeons of England in 1974. It appears that elevated temperature produces some kind of shock protein on cancer membranes and enabling immune system to identify this alien tissue.

Hyperthermia is usually achieved via exposure to warm blankets, air or by water in hot bath. It is applied for 1 hour daily for several months.

Diet

No small number of alternative practitioners ranging from Norman Walker to Lorraine Day identifies right diet as best cure against cancer. It usually consists of lots of vegetables, salads, sea weeds, fresh juices etc. It prohibits sugar and its derivates as well as all sorts of processed foods and often meat as well. What people don't usually know is that proper diet depends on particular blood type. For example blood type 0 is oldest blood type dating to time when people consumed exclusively meat. If placed on diet this blood type should still preserve some "healthy grown" meat on menu while other groups no. A, B are newer blood types and AB is merely few thousand years old. These blood types require more vegetables even without strict diet. Search the web for diets per blood types.

---

[65] http://www.thewolfeclinic.com/index.php/information-and-tools/protocols/136-the-cesium-chloride-protocol

III. CONCLUSION

Generally speaking, cancer issue is a very complex one. "Official" medicine usually has diametrically opposite views about what cancer is and how to treat it than "alternative" medicine and it's practitioners. And "official" medicine in USA is bit different than "official" medicine in Germany meaning German clinics often employ something that would be considered "alternative" medicine in USA. Why respective American institutions continue to ferociously ban alternative practices (which often report much higher patient "survival rates") remains a question of speculation. And all that is very relevant to cancer patients as humanity is supposed to "pool medical knowledge" in most effective way around the world and not protect it via everlasting patents or, even worse, suppress it.

Thankfully, modern technologies like internet enable synthesis of this knowledge. Taking that into account and going back to basics of what was said so far - when thinking of cancer we should not think of fear related to it but rather of things that are very relevant to it's existence like:

a) low oxygen environment

b) acidic body

c) excess glucose in blood

d) exposure to radiation

e) toxic build up in body

f) various parasites

It should be said that usually one reason alone is usually not enough to develop cancer. Causes are usually *self-amplifying* and *compounding*. Therefore one action alone is not enough to prevent or treat cancer. It can take several things to cause cancer and addressing each one of them in time reduces the *possibility* of cancer development. So in that way it is really the <u>question of risk management</u>. Raising the notch in one of mentioned areas raises your overall risk of developing cancer. And there is a threshold value when it will occur. People don't realize that it usually takes up to 4 years before detecting that cancer has developed.

Different people are also influenced by different causes or *levels* of different causes. If we quickly refer back to Chapter 1 and "Pillars of health" we can see that globally three categories mostly affects cancer development and that are: food, hazardous influence (radiation+infections) and state of our immune system. Person eating quality organic food, without exposure to significant radiation and toxins, somewhat slim and exercised is much less likely to develop cancer than person with opposite characteristics.

This book also revealed other maybe "forgotten" or "sidelined" issues in cancer development. Primarily we should mention Dr. Warburgs threshold of 35% oxygen reduction required to start cancerous process. Oxygen is absorbed from air and in cellular respiration converted with glucose to energy using coenzymeQ10. Acidity of body, polluted - oxygen starved air, food, obesity all play important role in cancer stage. Sugar related inhibition of immune system, acidic digestion, consequential obesity and suppression of "autophagy process" are of prime importance to cancer development.

From what was mentioned we can conclude that cancer (and its variants) is not yet thoroughly and scientifically researched to a point scientists can say exactly who will develop cancer and what methods will surely cure cancer as death rates are still very high. Fortunately "alternative" practitioners and abundance of simpler trial&error method have brought forward interesting and cheap ways of cancer prevention and treatment which were described in previous chapters.

This book overall should not be viewed as "alternative" medicine to cancer treatment. It merely points out some things that are not commonly known but does not, on any occasion, contravene elementary logic. "Official" methods of cancer treatment, especially surgery, is well justified in respective cases. For example if stomach&intestine cancer has grown few pounds in weight it is highly unlikely it will be cured by carrot juice or sodium bicarbonate. Surgery is most reasonable method to remove such mass of unnecessary tissue. Also in other cases when cancer is very small, a lump so to speak, it makes every sense to surgically remove it before it spreads around and not put all the eggs in "alternative" basket. There are no rules however prohibiting use of "alternative" treatments like juice diet, sodium bicarbonate, enzyme supplements, flax seed protocol etc. with official medicine (except in special cases). So patient at least can be satisfied it is doing all it possibly can.

"Alternative" practitioners cured thousands of people and there is no reason why you may not consider this approach - especially if everything else, including official medicine, fails.

Point of no return

As with many other things there is point of no return in cancer development. After this point is passed no surgery or cure in the world will help anymore. Therefore it is important to be conscious of it. But there are also some milestones before this point. For example every individual is exposed to some cancerous processes to a point you don't even see it. When cancer cells grow to few billions they become physically visible or sensible. The difference is whether the immune system is strong enough to handle it on time or not. If cancer obviously starts to develop there is usually limited timeframe for action. Many things influence cancer development and many things may influence it's remedy. And it is up to you "dear reader" to decide what action you will take and when.

In continuation I summarized important points for cancer prevention and treatment.

Prevention

You can do no wrong by doing the following:

1. Check pH value of your body every few months with saliva and urinary tests

2. Check where Curry and Hartman lines are in your apartment - crosses are most dangerous

3. Check level of electromagnetic radiation in your apartment

4. Eat more fresh vegetables and fruits and especially drink more fresh juice from your juicer

5. Cut down animal protein input (especially from non-organic origin)

6. Cut down input of sugar and it's derivates

7. Cut down input of carbohydrates

8. Clean your bowels thoroughly (using magnesium salt) and feast for 2 days[66] every 6 months

9. Remove stressors from your life

10. Avoid highly processed and canned food and all sorts of soda. Drink natural lemonade instead.

11. Eat more alkaline food, if your pH is lower than 6.5 drink sodium bicarbonate [67] (from drugstore)

12. Eat more antioxidants related food as measured in ORAC scale

13. Cut down input of cow milk and dairy products

14. Achieve "inner peace" to alleviate stress either by spending time in nature or by other means. Your soul must be at ease and rested from depressing thoughts

15. Get good night's sleep for at least 7 hours daily

16. Consume supplements of unsaturated fatty acids (Omega 3-6-9) and enzyme CoQ10

17. Filter chlorine from water

18. Apply flax seed, diet, fresh juice, sodium bicarbonate, Aloe Vera protocols as prescribed from time to time

19. Perform regular and moderate physical exercise in fresh air (like jogging 30 min. each day)

21. Avoid excess use of fluoridated tooth paste

22. Dump all teflon cookware immediately

23. Watch out for harmful E additives in food as mentioned earlier in text

24. Take supplemental pancreatic enzymes

Underlying concept of all stuff listed above comes down to three basic and logical things:

    a)   eat nutritious food that your body can really use, not junk
    b)   avoid toxins, stress and all sort of radiation
    c)   perform regular detoxification, exercise and give your body a chance to heal itself.

---

[66] Person at risk will obviously skip this point

[67] People at risk from intake of soda bicarbonate will obviously skip this point

Treatment

Unfortunately for people diagnosed with advanced and aggressive forms of cancer there is less to be done but one should never give up hope. For early cancer patients, however there is no reason for pessimism and advices provided above are hugely beneficial. However, if you feel that it isn't enough and you think official medical treatment is not helping you, you can take additional measures:

1. All things mentioned in above mentioned "Prevention"

2. Severely reduce input of animal protein, carbohydrates, dairy products

3. Monthly cleansing of bowels combined with daily input of 2 liters of fresh vegetables juice

4. Carry out instant alkalization by drinking daily three glasses of soda bicarbonate (from

   drugstore) until pH is over 7

5. Stop all input of all sugar, sodas, processed and canned food

6. Try some or all other mentioned alternative protocols. Beware though, cesium protocol is dangerous in you exceed cesium level or drop below required level of potassium. Bob Beck protocol should not be mixed with other protocols.

You must be aware that you take these somewhat extreme steps on your own responsibility and authors or publisher may not be held responsible for any resulting liability or event. These are merely the things that sometimes helped people when all else has failed.

What is interesting is that after writing this book I noticed that number of these points is similar to guidelines issued by American Cancer Society Guidelines[68] regarding concerning diet, feasting, sugar intake and exercise.

Highlights

I choose this subchapter as to flash few rough but maybe unknown facts for eager readers:

- 1.6 million man in USA are expected be diagnosed with cancer in 2012[69]
- Patents exist on cheap cures for HIV and cancer
- Only 10% of cancer cases are of hereditary nature
- Most cancer cases are easily preventable
- Body acidity significantly affects cancer development
- Sugar (glucose) severely inhibits immune system (up to 75% reduction in neutrophil activity)
- Cancer cells lost their advanced primary function of specialized work and returned to primitive form of multiplication for sheer survival
- Cancer cells produce energy anaerobically - without oxygen
- They produce energy with 20 times lower efficiency than normal cells thereby devouring glucose and other protein mass (patients loose weight)

[68] http://onlinelibrary.wiley.com/doi/10.3322/caac.20140/full

[69] American Cancer Society; Cancer fact&figures report 2012

- Cancer cells have 10 times more insulin receptors than normal ones
- Cells can turn cancerous when starved of oxygen (Dr. Warburg won Nobel prize in 1931 for this discovery)
- Acidity of human body depends also on type of food and water intake
- Pathogenic Hartman and Curry lines can lead to cancer
- Feasting stimulates autophagy process that clears "junk" from human body
- Average animal meat aside useful proteins includes growth hormones, pesticides, antibiotics which can be mutagens
- Cow milk is rich in casein and it's digestion produces lots of slime lots of bacteria
- Chlorine in drinking water is pesticide
- Clogged up colon is toxic and causes many diseases including cancer
- Stress induces cortisol which suppresses the immune response
- Sodium bicarbonate, strongly alkalizes body and destroys Candida Albicans - suspect cause of cancer
- Because of artificial sweeteners (aspartame) „0%" sugar sodas are usually much more dangerous than sugar ones
- According to one study, most oncologists would refuse chemotherapy as method of treatment[70]

---

[70] According to 1986 survey carried out in at McGill University of chemotherapy drugs for lung cancer.

Useful links:

Independent Cancer Research Foundation

http://www.cancertutor.com

International Agency for Research on Cancer

http://www.iarc.fr/

World Cancer Research Fund International

http://www.wcrf.org/

National Cancer Institute

http://www.cancer.gov

American Cancer Society

http://www.cancer.org/

About.com Cancer

http://cancer.about.com/od/

National Center for Biotechnology Information

http://www.ncbi.nlm.nih